Men's Health

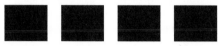

Life Improvement Guides®

Healing Power

Natural Methods
for Achieving
Whole-Body Health

by Bridget Doherty, Doug Hill,
and the Editors of **Men'sHealth** Books

Rodale Press, Inc.
Emmaus, Pennsylvania

Copyright © 1999 by Rodale Press, Inc.

Illustrations copyright © 1999 by Alan Baseden and Bryon Thompson

All rights reserved. No part of this publication may be reproduced or transmitted in any form or by any means, electronic or mechanical, including photocopying, recording, or any other information storage and retrieval system, without the written permission of the publisher.

Men's Health Books and *Men's Health Life Improvement Guides* are registered trademarks of Rodale Press, Inc.

Printed in the United States of America on acid-free ♾, recycled paper ♲

Other titles in the *Men's Health Life Improvement Guides* series:

Command Respect	*Food Smart*	*Money Savvy*	*Stress Blasters*	*Vitamin Vitality*
Death Defiers	*Good Loving*	*Powerfully Fit*	*Stronger Faster*	
Fight Fat	*Maximum Style*	*Sex Secrets*	*Symptom Solver*	

Library of Congress Cataloging-in-Publication Data

Doherty, Bridget.
    Healing power : natural methods for achieving whole-body health /
by Bridget Doherty, Doug Hill, and the editors of Men's Health
Books.
        p.   cm. — (Men's health life improvement guides)
    Includes index.
    ISBN 0–87596–506–7 paperback
    1. Men—Health and hygiene.   2. Alternative medicine.   I. Hill,
Doug, 1950– . II. Men's Health Books. III. Title. IV. Series.
RA777.8.D63   1999
613'.04234—dc21   98–48717

Distributed to the book trade by St. Martin's Press

2   4   6   8   10   9   7   5   3   1   paperback

—— OUR PURPOSE ——

*"We inspire and enable people to improve
their lives and the world around them."*

Healing Power Staff

Managing Editor: **Jack Croft**

Senior Editor: **Stephen C. George**

Writers: **Bridget Doherty, Doug Hill**

Contributing Writers: **Erik D'Amato, Grete Haentjens, Lois Guarino Hazel, Deanna Moyer, Lorna S. Sapp**

Associate Research Manager: **Jane Unger Hahn**

Lead Researcher: **Lorna S. Sapp**

Editorial Researchers: **Jennifer Abel, Carol J. Gilmore, Mary S. Mesaros, Deanna Moyer, Paula Rasich, Staci Ann Sander, Shea Zukowski**

Copy Editors: **Kathryn A. Cressman, David R. Umla**

Associate Art Director: **Charles Beasley**

Cover Designer and Series Art Director: **Tanja Lipinski-Cole**

Series Designer: **John Herr**

Cover Photographer: **Mitch Mandel**

Cover Hand Model: **Jennifer A. Barefoot**

Part Opener Illustrator: **Alan Baseden**

Chapter Opener Illustrator: **Bryon Thompson**

Layout Designer: **Donna G. Rossi**

Manufacturing Coordinator: **Melinda B. Rizzo**

Office Manager: **Roberta Mulliner**

Office Staff: **Julie Kehs, Mary Lou Stephen**

Rodale Health and Fitness Books

Vice President and Editorial Director: **Debora T. Yost**

Executive Editor: **Neil Wertheimer**

Design and Production Director: **Michael Ward**

Marketing Manager: **Sharon Lawler-Sudell**

Research Manager: **Ann Gossy Yermish**

Copy Manager: **Lisa D. Andruscavage**

Production Manager: **Robert V. Anderson Jr.**

Associate Studio Manager: **Thomas P. Aczel**

Manufacturing Managers: **Eileen F. Bauder, Mark Krahforst**

Photo Credits

Page 152: **Judy Katz Public Relations**

Page 154: **U. S. Senator Tom Harkin**

Page 156: **Mike Ridewood/Canadian Olympic Association**

Page 158: **Oscar Janiger, M.D.**

Back flap: **Hulton Getty/Liason Agency Inc.**

Contents

Part Five
Real-Life Scenarios

Quest for the Best

You Can Do It!

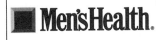

Introduction

Power to the People

By 1994, U2 was just about the biggest rock band in the world. Their technologically dazzling and musically daring Zoo TV Tour sold out arenas and stadiums throughout North America and Europe, and their records sold in the millions. So it was hardly a surprise that their 1993 release, *Zooropa*, won a Grammy Award. What did seem more than a little odd, though, was that it won for Best Alternative Album.

Only in the eyes of the staid recording-industry establishment could one of rock's biggest money-makers be seen as "alternative." The award left even the Irish band's lead singer, Bono, shaking his head. If U2 was "alternative," what, precisely, was "mainstream"?

The medical establishment faces a similar question today. And just as in the music world, the line between what's considered "alternative" and "mainstream" has blurred to the point where it's often tough to tell which is which.

Now, if you're like me, you may be more than a little skeptical about anything carrying the tag line "alternative," especially when it comes to health. The only Yogi I ever thought was worth following lives in Jellystone Park, has a fondness for picnic baskets, and is worshipped by just one disciple, known as Boo-Boo.

But do I consider myself a man who is open to alternatives? Absolutely. To my mind, being alternative simply means believing there's more than one way of doing things. That's especially true where your health in concerned. Don't get me wrong: I have great respect for conventional medicine and the doctors who take care of us, but I don't believe they're the last word on my well-being. I'm the last word.

And this is a book about the other ways of doing things. Yes, *Healing Power* is a user's manual of alternative medicine. Alternative in the sense that it's a guide to something other than sweating it out in a waiting room; something besides letting a person in a white coat make you feel powerless and meek;

something instead of invasive, side-effect-riddled procedures and pharmaceuticals.

It's about adventure. Anyone can buy a pill and swallow it, but it takes a certain kind of man to uncover the secret wisdom and healing remedies of an ancient civilization and then be daring enough to try those remedies to cure his own ailments.

It's about knowledge, which means, of course, that it's also about power. Don't believe it? Imagine two men side by side. Both have headaches. One guy knows just one way to get rid of it: Take an aspirin. But the other guy knows all the other ways, including four herbs and a special oil that are all just as strong as aspirin, plus five different pressure points that melt pain as soon as you touch them. Who has more power?

It's about control. In this book, you'll learn to not only take charge of your health but also to yoke the very power of nature itself for your own personal use.

Finally, it's about the thrill of exploration. As you'll see, alternative medicine is a whole new world, an exotic landscape that you get to uncover, whose secrets you get to bring back and use in your own world. To soothe everyday aches and pains. To block stress. To keep your heart healthy. To make your sex life more exciting. To make your life more enjoyable. To make you more powerful.

In the end, all "alternative" means is that you get to learn about all the other options. Different options, sure. Unusual options, almost certainly. And, quite possibly, better options. And that could only make you, in the words of a very wise Yogi, "smarter than the average bear."

Jack Croft

Jack Croft
Managing Editor, *Men's Health* Books

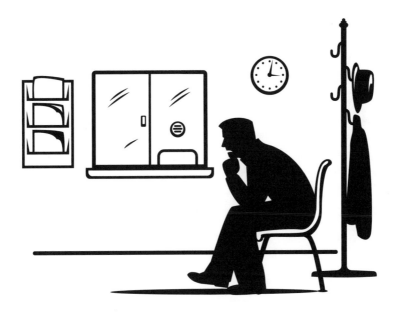

Part One

A Whole World of Healing

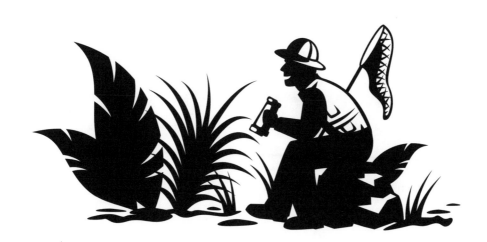

Taking Control of Your Health

Discovering Brave New Worlds

Where men stand today in American health care is where the *voyageurs* must have stood centuries ago when they began exploring the inland frontier of early America. Up ahead, a whole new world of exotic unknown wonder and mystery lies in wait. It's big and tantalizingly beautiful but also alien and strange. Behind—where we've come from—sit all of the traditions and practices and laws of the Old World.

You have two choices. You can turn around as fast as possible and hightail it back to familiar territory. Or you can become an explorer.

For us today, that vast, undiscovered country ahead is alternative medicine: acupuncture, herbal therapy, homeopathy, massage therapy, naturopathy—the whole range of options we're going to explore in this book. The Old World consists entirely of a doctor's office, a drugstore, and a hospital. If you get sick, call the doctor. He'll tell you what to do.

In the new era of health care, the ways of the old system are over. Today, as never before, we can become active participants in taking care of our own health. There are myriad options available that don't involve taking pills or undergoing surgery. We learn how to use those options, not only to avoid becoming sick in the first place but also to achieve a greater state of wellness than we've ever imagined possible.

That's the world envisioned by people like Robert Ivker, D.O., president of the American Holistic Medical Association, co-author of the book *Thriving: The Holistic Guide to Optimal Health for Men*, and a holistic family physician in Littleton, Colorado. "Each of us has the capacity to heal himself," he says. "It's really about becoming more conscious—heightening our awareness of our bodies, minds, and spirits so that we can do the things that enhance the condition of all three. What makes our bodies feel vital? What gives our bodies health and energy? What depletes that energy? That takes a higher level of awareness than most men have developed about themselves up to this point."

Options Unlimited

That lack of awareness is changing, Dr. Ivker believes, in part because men are learning that they have more options and in part because they are realizing how important it is to their own health and well-beings to seek out new options. That's so for several reasons. It's becoming increasingly obvious, for one, that conventional medicine has limits: The men and women in white coats don't have all the answers. And the options they do have available—drugs and surgery, for the most part—can debilitate as well as cure. It's better, we see now, to live in such a way that these desperate rescue measures won't be needed. It's also better to have other less drastic alternatives to use as first resorts.

In addition, and perhaps most important of all, research is making it abundantly clear that the more we participate in taking care of our own health, the healthier we are likely to be. Attitude counts: an active, involved, positive attitude promotes physical well-being. "Being dependent not only makes you dependent, which a lot of guys don't like, but also often doesn't work," says James S. Gordon, M.D., director of the Center for Mind/Body Medicine in Washington, D.C.

In his book *Manifesto for a New Medicine: Your Guide to Healing Partnerships and the Wise Use of Alternative Therapies*, Dr. Gordon calls for a "healing partnership" between patient and doctor. "My responsibility is to help people to discover for themselves what is best for them," he writes. "I'm there to share my knowledge and whatever wisdom I may have, and to help them understand their lives and explore their options."

Alternative medicine in general is far more oriented toward preventing illness and optimizing health than conventional medicine has traditionally been. The problem is that much of this huge new territory is relatively uncharted. HMOs and insurance companies won't, in most cases, take you there. Many doctors know little or nothing about it. It's up to each of us to find his own way.

New World Resources

The good news is that there are vast new sources of health care information opening up that can help you navigate. Books like this one are part of the publishing industry's response to a huge consumer demand for information on alternative forms of health care. That same demand is reflected in a mega-explosion of health care information on the Internet. If information is power, then power over health care decisions in this country is clearly shifting out of the grip of the few and into the hands of the many.

One doctor who studies this shift is Tom Ferguson, M.D., a senior associate at the Center for Clinical Computing in Boston and author of the book *Health Online*. "Online, you see people defining their own ideas of what represents quality information. The consumers are increasingly making the choices," he says.

This emerging new paradigm is most clear, Dr. Ferguson believes, in the thousands of health care discussion groups that have blossomed on the Internet, where people gather to trade experiences and information on specific conditions with which they or their loved ones are afflicted. These groups represent a huge mechanism for gathering and pooling information. Not all of the information on display there is reliable, to be sure.

"You can't check your brain at the door," Dr. Ferguson says. But, in most cases, off-the-wall claims don't go unchallenged by other members of the group, and medical doctors who specialize in a particular area often participate in the discussions, helping to filter out misinformation.

The result is an unprecedented empowerment of the individual consumer, Dr. Ferguson says. Patients who used to wait for their doctors to explain to them what was happening with their condition and what could be done about it now arrive in their doctors' offices with literally hundreds of pages of information downloaded from the Internet. "This new technology will demand a major role change for most doctors—from unquestioned gurus to partners and collaborators," Dr. Ferguson says.

Not all doctors greet empowered patients enthusiastically, although there are signs that that is changing. The title of an address delivered to the 1996 annual meeting of the American Medical Association was "Debunking the Myth about Health Care: Put the Patient in the Driver's Seat." The Association's president, Daniel H. Johnson Jr., M.D., spoke in the strongest terms about "the one myth that disturbs me the most—the notion that patients are too stupid to make decisions for themselves."

Whether a given doctor is ready to become a collaborator rather than the sole decision-maker isn't the real issue, though. You can always find another doctor. Given that the locus of health care control is shifting to the patient, the real question is directed at you.

Are you ready to go exploring?

Healing through History

Recapturing Ancient Wisdom

In 1971, the appendix of *New York Times* columnist James Reston earned a small but distinctive footnote in the annals of American medicine.

Reston's appendix burst while he was on a visit to China with then head of the National Security Council Henry Kissinger. It was on this trip that Kissinger finalized plans for President Richard Nixon's historic visit to China the following year. Reston decided to try the ancient healing method of acupuncture instead of drugs to help relieve some of his postoperative pain.

In those days, Reston was the very embodiment of mainstream journalism, as level-headed as they come. If he said there was something to this acupuncture stuff, well, that was news. And indeed, Reston became a believer. His account of the experience—"a man publishing an obituary notice on his own appendix," he sardonically called it—appeared on the front page of the *Times* 10 days later.

Reston didn't utterly abandon his reportorial skepticism—he took due note of the communist political slogans that were prominently posted in the hospital—but he left no doubt that something extraordinary had occurred. The treatment was exotic, mysterious, and inexplicable by Western standards. It was also quite effective.

In the years since Reston's epiphany, a lot of Americans have been looking at the healing wisdom of the past and

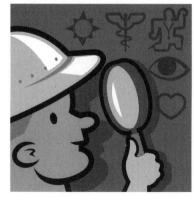

discovering that it works. Nonetheless, many people still see alternative medicine as the new kid on the health care block. That's ironic because if there's anything new in health care, it's the high-tech approach that most of us take for granted when we walk into our doctors' offices.

Consider the following dates.

- The first x-ray of human bones was taken in 1896. By the 1950s, more than half the general practitioners in the United States still didn't have an x-ray machine.
- By the start of World War II, penicillin was still in the laboratory stage. Diseases such as meningitis, tuberculosis, and polio were still often fatal.
- Open-heart surgery dates from the 1950s; bypass operations began in 1967.

Compare those dates to these.

- Ayurveda, India's "science of life," is based on ancient Hindu texts some 5,000 years old.
- Acupuncture was described at length by China's Yellow Emperor around 2600 B.C. It is derived from traditions that had been transmitted orally for many centuries before that.

Just because a treatment is old doesn't mean that it's good, of course. We're grateful that hemorrhoids are no longer being cauterized with a red-hot iron, and we don't particularly miss bloodletting, either. But not all the knowledge of our ancestors was ignorance and superstition, not by a long shot.

"What we call medicine today is very limited," says Douglas Schar, a practicing herbalist in London and author of *The Backyard Medicine Chest.* "In the past, the tapestry was much richer. Diet, nutrition, herbs, exercise, prayer— they were all used as a matter of course. Healing was mental, physical, and spiritual. That held true up until about 1920, when everything started to come out of a test tube. Science and technology took over. What we're doing is simply getting back to what has always been."

With that mission in mind, here's a quick tour through the history of healing, from an alternative point of view.

Harmony and Energy

Human efforts to heal ourselves are as old as the diseases that afflict us. A fragment of carved reindeer rib dating from 30,000 B.C. shows a Paleolithic shaman in an animal mask—a healer—performing a ceremonial dance. Skulls that show evidence of having been pierced by surgeons date back at least 10,000 years. Anthropologists suspect that these primitive operations were intended to release evil spirits, perhaps from tribesmen plagued by mental illness or epilepsy. Whether they were successful on that score is unknown, but it's apparent from the condition of the skulls that the surgical incisions healed.

Health and religion have been intimately connected since ancient times. Holy men and healers were often the same person; in Greece, temples for the gods were also health spas. The words *holiness* and *healing*, in fact, stem from a common root. Good health was seen as being in tune with the forces of nature, while illness was the result of some imbalance of those same forces. This idea, which is a central belief of many alternative healers today, surfaces in sources as distant from one another as China's *Tao-te Ching*, written in the sixth cen-

The Royal Treatment

"Help, or at least do no harm," Hippocrates said, and most practitioners of alternative medicine are proud of how gentle and harmless their treatments are. But "natural" medicine has been practiced pretty aggressively in days gone by, as authors Robert Buckman, Ph.D., and Karl Sabbagh demonstrate in their book *Magic or Medicine?: An Investigation of Healing and Healers*. They provide the following account of how physicians tried to revive Britain's King Charles II after he collapsed in 1685.

"The king was bled to the extent of a pint from a vein in his right arm. Next, his shoulder was cut into, and the incised area was supped to suck out an additional eight ounces of blood. An emetic and a purgative were administered followed by a second purgative followed by an enema containing antimony, sacred bitters, rock salt, mallow leaves, violets, beetroot, chamomile flowers, fennel seed, linseed, cinnamon, cardamom seed, saffron, cochineal, and aloes. The king's scalp was shaved and a blister raised. A sneezing powder of hellebore was administered. A plaster of Burgundy pitch and pigeon dung was applied to the feet. Medicaments included melon seeds, manna, slippery elm, black cherry water, lime flowers, lily of the valley, peony, lavender, and dissolved pearls. As he grew worse, 40 drops of extract of human skull were administered followed by a rallying dose of Raleigh's antidote."

Curiously, the authors report, the king's strength seemed to wane after these interventions. Other equally heroic measures also failed, and His Majesty expired.

tury B.C., and the observations of the Greek physician Hippocrates, as recorded by a variety of authors in the *Corpus Hippocraticcum* in the fourth century B.C. For Hippocrates, the goal of healing was to help the body attain a state of harmony, at which point it would heal itself.

A related concept that emerges with startling consistency across the ages is the idea that some type of energy or life force is a necessary component of health. This, too, has been embraced by alternative healers. "Virtually all the fields of alternative medicine have the idea of subtle energies at their base," says David Edelberg, M.D., chairman and founder of American WholeHealth, a holistic health center in Chicago. "In Chinese medicine, it's called *chi* (pronounced chee); in Ayurveda, it's *prana*; in Japan, it's *ki*. Homeopaths call it the vital force, chiropractors call it innate energy, and naturopaths refer to *vis medicatrix naturae*, which is Latin for 'the healing power of nature.' Conventional doctors don't understand this, but I find that patients intuitively do. It's not something that you can measure."

The idea of preserving or re-aligning this natural energy is one reason that holistic practitioners try to take a man's complete health picture—diet, exercise, and mental, emotional, and spiritual conditions—into account. Even back in ancient Greece, it was standard, if informal, medical procedure.

In the Beginning, We Ate

The first health regimen was food, and sticking to it was relatively simple: For Stone Age man, nothing but "natural" products were available. The foods our prehistoric ancestors regularly consumed provided half the fat of modern diets, twice the calcium, 5 to 10 times the amount of fiber, a quarter of the salt, no alcohol, and hardly any sugar, says S. Boyd Eaton, M.D., associate clinical professor of radiology and adjunct associate professor of anthropology at Emory University in Atlanta and co-author of *The Paleolithic Prescription*. Our bodies literally evolved on that kind of nutritional balance, he says, and by eating any differently, we're going against our genetic

natures. That helps explain why "diseases of civilization" such as cancer, heart disease, high blood pressure, and obesity only became common in modern times.

Foods that were dangerous were known in antiquity, too. Witness the prohibitions against pork and shellfish in the Old Testament. "The dietary laws in Leviticus were intended to be a prescription for health from God to the Israelites," says Schar. "And, in fact, if you followed the rules, you were less likely to become ill."

Roots and Greens

In prehistory, there were no all-night drugstores. So where would a caveman turn if he was feeling punkish? Almost certainly to an herbalist or directly to the herbs themselves. Zoologists have identified as many as eight species of primates that use plants for medicinal purposes, according to James A. Duke, Ph.D., a botanist retired from the U.S. Department of Agriculture and author of *The Green Pharmacy*. "If the apes can figure it out, I guess humans can, too," he says.

The discovery in Iraq of the 60,000-year-old remains of a primitive man also suggests that we were using herbal remedies quite early in our evolutionary career, Dr. Duke adds: The gentleman was carrying seven varieties of healing herbs, among them ephedra, a powerful stimulant and decongestant. Today, you know its chemical stepbrother as Sudafed.

Modern Times

Most historians place the dawning of modern medicine around the sixteenth century, although they'll quibble over which invention or idea represents the crucial breakthrough. René Descartes's separation of mind and body is often mentioned as the wedge that drove religion and medicine apart, while Francis Bacon's advocacy of inductive reasoning is said to have ushered in the age of objective science. A new precision in anatomical drawing, together with the growing acceptability of dissecting human corpses for medical research, opened the way for huge advances in understanding how the body works. That knowledge, in turn, was filtered through Isaac Newton's vision of a clockwork universe. The human body, like the planets, was now seen as an assembly of systems that ran according to the mechanical laws of physics. Suddenly, we had come a long way from shamans dancing around with antlers on their heads.

The microscope may be the best symbol of the dramatic perceptual shift that occurred at the beginning of the modern era. Invented as early as the late 1500s, it wasn't until the 1840s that microscopes were technically refined enough to become an effective research tool. At that point, everything changed. Most of the medical miracles of the twentieth century—bacteriology, pharmacology, immunology, neurobiology, and genetics, to name a few—derive from the access we gained to the microscopic world.

But that fantastic voyage into the interior narrowed medicine's focus radically. As scientists peered ever more intently at tissues and cells, the holistic view, which sees each of us as intimately connected to his environment, to other people, to the universe, to God, was lost. And the human factor began to disappear with it. "Doctors directed their gazes not on the individual sick person but on the disease of which his body was the bearer," writes Roy Porter, Ph.D., professor in the social history of medicine at the Wellcome Institute in London and editor of *The Cambridge Illustrated History of Medicine.*

This shift within science coincided with an equally momentous shift in society as a whole: the Industrial Revolution. Millions of citi-

The Future: Flush with Excitement

Where will medicine go from here? Holistic, natural healing practices may flourish, but that doesn't mean high-tech health care is going away. Genetic engineering alone may revolutionize preventive medicine by allowing us to replace defective genes before they cause disease, while drugs designed by computers could just as thoroughly revolutionize pharmacology.

For sheer convenience, though, it will be hard to beat a new diagnostic tool predicted by some Japanese researchers: the intelligent toilet. This superjohn will monitor urine and feces for the presence of blood, sugar, and other substances. Results will be dispatched via telephone line to a central computerized monitoring system. If a problem is detected, the, uh, depositor would be notified and encouraged to see a doctor.

zens were leaving their farms for the cities, where they lost touch, literally, with the natural foods and herbs that had surrounded them. "At the turn of the century, most of the American population lived in a rural setting," says Schar. "Today, most people live in or near a city. As that shift took place, people became dependent on what they could get in a store." The era of instant pizza and the 12-hour cold capsule was just around the corner.

After 100 years of urban living, how connected are we to the natural remedies that sustained our forefathers? Not very. About the only herb many Americans could identify today is marijuana. Our health has suffered, in many cases, from that loss, which is why alternative practitioners are urging us to take a giant step backward, not as an exercise in nostalgia but so that we can once again take a look at the bigger picture.

Conventional versus Natural Medicine

When Worlds Collide

Here's a true story: A scientist who believes passionately in the benefits of alternative therapies was trying for the thousandth time to convince his best friend, a successful general practitioner, to at least consider using them. At one point, the general practitioner cut off the discussion.

"You don't seem to get it," he told his scientist friend. "I didn't go to medical school and spend 25 years practicing medicine to sit with my patients and tell them what they should eat for breakfast."

For anyone involved in alternative medicine, that comment explains perfectly how conventional health care has lost its grip on reality. Most medical doctors, alternative practitioners believe, are addicted to the "big fix": strong drugs, supersophisticated technology, and major surgery.

Alternative medicine today is challenging the assumption that the big fix is the safest, cheapest, and best way to keep people well. But that's just one of the sacred medical cows that it's taking on.

Emergencies Aren't Everything

No one is saying that there aren't many things that conventional medicine does extremely well. The point is that it doesn't necessarily do everything well. "Western medicine

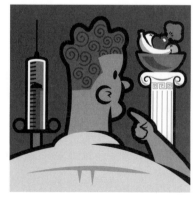

has made its greatest mark in taking care of severe, acute problems," says M. Kyu Chung, M.D., a certified acupuncturist and chief of family medicine at Cooper Health Systems in Camden, New Jersey. "Trauma cases, heart attacks, cancer cases in which surgery is the best treatment: Those are the sorts of things that Western medicine handles best because it tends to focus on disease. Where Western medicine has largely failed is in taking care of the more chronic conditions, things like arthritis, back pain, neck pain, headache, bowel disease, and fatigue disorders. Alternative medicine does better with those sorts of problems because there's much more attention paid to keeping people well, consistently, over time."

Indeed, promoting overall "wellness" is a fundamental orientation of holistic medicine. Dr. Chung says that in China, people traditionally paid their doctors to keep them healthy; when they got sick, they stopped paying. While alternative practitioners in this country will presumably skip the no-payment option, there's no question that they've followed the Chinese emphasis on prevention and on treating the whole person rather than a specific disease.

Gentle Healing

Alternative practitioners also make a point of trying to find the gentlest possible treatment for any health problem they encounter. One reason the alternative movement is growing so rapidly, they say, is that the public has become increasingly fearful of the debilitating side effects that so often accompany conventional treatments. Those fears are well-founded, according to Bruce Pomeranz, M.D., Ph.D., a neurophysiologist at the University of Toronto Medical School and a leading researcher into the physiological effects of acupuncture. "When you examine the death rates for drugs and surgery, you fall off your chair," he says. "We're killing people with procedures that may not even work. I've shown that properly prescribed drugs killed 106,000 Americans in 1994. So when you ask whether there's any role for alternative medicine, there's your answer: Why take drastic measures when you can try safer measures first?"

That's the alternative approach in a nutshell: Always begin with the least invasive treatment and then, when necessary, go up the ladder from there. A patient with rheumatoid arthritis, for example, might get a treatment plan that starts with a detoxifying diet of raw fruits and vegetables, says Dr. James S. Gordon of the Center for Mind/Body Medicine. Next on the list would be regular acupuncture treatments to reduce inflammation, and yoga classes to restore flexibility and motion. Herbs that soothe frozen joints might also be prescribed, along with meditation exercises to reduce stress. Prescription drugs and surgery would be last resorts, adds Dr. Gordon.

An important corollary of this approach is that the less invasive the treatment, the less it's likely to cost, says Dr. David Edelberg of American WholeHealth. A lot of insurance companies are becoming surprisingly progressive on the issue of alternative health care for the simple reason that visits to a yoga instructor tend to be cheaper—a lot cheaper—than visits to a heart surgeon.

The Personal Touch

One of the most important differences between alternative and conventional health care is the amount of time and attention devoted to patients. A visit to a holistic practitioner can last an hour or more, especially for

---

A Report from the Front

Is there any hope that the American medical establishment will begin to take alternative medicine seriously? Yes, but it won't happen overnight, say doctors who have been advocating the advantages of alternative therapies for years.

For example, Dr. David Edelberg of American WholeHealth edited an encyclopedia of alternative medicine for the American Medical Association, only to see it shoved under the table. "They decided that it was too controversial for the membership," he said.

Still, there are signs of change. One of them can be detected in the growing number of conventional medical schools that include alternative medicine in their curricula. Figures compiled by the Association of American Medical Colleges show that in the 1996–97 school year, 60 schools covered alternative medicine in required courses and 56 offered elective classes on it.

For advocates of holistic health care, that's progress. Skeptics could point out, however, that, as of 1997, no American medical school offered a required course strictly on alternative medicine.

---

the first session, says Dr. Edelberg. And that's time spent with the doctor, not reading magazines in the waiting room. Alternative therapists don't keep a leisurely pace just because they're chatty. How a patient feels emotionally, psychologically, and spiritually has a major impact, they believe, on the way he feels physically. "In conventional medicine, diagnosis and treatment are like the socks you buy at Kmart: one size fits all," says Dr. Edelberg. "In holistic medicine, the goal is to determine how one's biography influences one's biology." The first thing Dr. Edelberg usually says to a new patient is "Tell me about the last time you felt fine."

Holistic practitioners also spend more time with their patients because they want the patients to participate in their own health care. The theory is that participation promotes self-healing. "Naturopaths believe that the patient is the healer," says Sheila Quinn, executive director of the American Association of Naturopathic Physicians in Seattle.

Doctor as Deity

The idea that doctors know best is deeply ingrained in our culture. So the concept that patients might have something to say about their own treatment seems like a radical and, to some, threatening notion. Indeed, alternative practitioners are convinced that it is the imperious and impersonal attitude that patients sometimes encounter in conventional health care that is driving them out of mainstream medicine.

Alternative practitioners love to point out that the real-life doctor behind the curtain is a lot more human than his infallible image would have us believe. Conventional medicine, they argue, is based a lot less on scientific research and a lot more on folklore and tradition than it likes to pretend. No one has ever proven how aspirin cures a headache, for example, but we rely on it quite comfortably just the same. Similarly, the factual foundations of conventional medical practice are by no means carved in stone: It's often said that about 50 percent of what any student learns in medical school will eventually be proven false. "When I think back to my medical school days, I wince," Dr. Edelberg says.

Nor does modern medical technology seem quite as invincible as it used to. A long list of diseases—AIDS, cancer, arthritis, Alzheimer's, colitis, diabetes, and multiple sclerosis, to name a few—have proved stubbornly resistant to cures, while new strains of bacteria have evolved, which are outwitting the best antibiotics we can throw at them. Alternative practi-

tioners believe that conventional doctors are becoming more receptive to holistic methods today because they are being forced to acknowledge that the big fix has limits.

Integrating the Two Systems

The goal of most alternative practitioners is not to beat conventional medicine but to join it. They talk of a complementary or integrative health care system, in part because they're willing to recognize their own limits. Not many advocates of holistic medicine would recommend that you report to a massage therapist when you think you're having a heart attack or when you need a liver transplant. They do envision and optimistically expect that the day will come when medical doctors will refer patients to herbalists, homeopaths, and acupuncturists as routinely as they make referrals now to dermatologists and physical therapists.

This optimism is based on three key observations. First, the economic strains of the current medical system are forcing a change toward more preventive, less invasive health care. Second, holistic practitioners say that many younger doctors seem more receptive to alternative methods than their older colleagues. Third, the general public is already leading a massive shift toward alternative therapies, whether the medical establishment likes it or not. "It's coming from the man on the street," says Dr. Pomeranz. "He's getting helped, his sister is getting helped, his uncle was helped, and they just keep going back."

Whether an integrated American health care system comes sooner or later is less certain, alternative's advocates say. Dr. Chung, for one, believes that it may come sooner. "Two years ago, I wouldn't have thought so, but now I'm not so sure."

Why the change?

"Because a significant number of my acupuncture patients are physicians' wives," Dr. Chung says. And even physicians themselves.

The Mind-Body Connection

What You Feel Affects How You Feel

No doubt, you've heard that you are what you eat. True enough, but that's not the whole story. You're also what you think and what you feel. What goes on between your ears has a major impact on what happens with the rest of your body, and vice versa.

On the surface, that statement may seem like simple common sense, but its implications are revolutionary. An avalanche of research in the past 20 to 30 years has shown that the mind and the body are far more intimately connected than we ever imagined, and those discoveries are at the heart of the challenge that alternative health care is posing to conventional medicine. "The research shows that what goes on in the mind as mediated through the emotions can affect every system and every organ of the body," says Dr. James S. Gordon of the Center for Mind/Body Medicine. "It's very exciting and very hopeful."

Emotional Molecules

Not so long ago, the science community believed that the mind and the immune system operated relatively independently of one another. We now know that that assumption was false. Researchers have discovered that there are nerves that connect the immune system to the nervous system, which, in turn, is directly wired to the brain. They have also discovered neuropeptides, molecules that carry messages between the brain and the immune system—to every cell in your body, in fact—enabling them to communicate constantly with one another.

Numerous experiments have verified the effects of this chemical exchange. One study, conducted at Ohio State University in Columbus, showed that students have poorer immune function during final exams. Another study, conducted at the University of California, Los Angeles, found that actors could cause changes in their immune systems merely by experiencing happiness or sadness when asked to think of specific scenarios.

What this means is that emotions can have a direct impact on the body's defenses against disease, theoretically making us more or less susceptible to everything from the common cold to AIDS. "The mental is physical, and the physical is mental," says Candace Pert, Ph.D., research professor of physiology and biophysics at Georgetown University Medical Center in Washington, D.C., and author of the book *Molecules of Emotion: Why You Feel the Way You Feel.* "The mind and the body are really inseparable. They're one."

From the Lab to the Streets

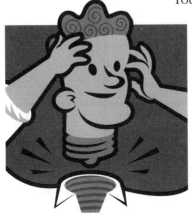

You don't have to look through a microscope in a laboratory to see the truth of the mind-body connection: Researchers have come to identical conclusions by observing thousands of men and women in the real world. One of the first such studies to gain widespread attention was the identification in the 1960s of the famous type A personality. Two California cardiologists demonstrated that type A men—those who were hurried, competitive, and hostile—were twice as likely to develop heart disease as men who didn't have those characteristics were. Subsequent researchers would refine that hypothesis, singling out hostility as the most unhealthy of the type A character traits.

In one study, some 1,300 men in Boston were given a questionnaire designed to determine their predispositions for anger. Possible responses included statements such as "At times, I feel like picking a fistfight" and "I have been so angry that I felt as if I would explode." Those whose test scores were highest were found to be three times more likely to develop heart disease than those with low scores were.

Hostility is harmful because it kicks off the fight-or-flight reflex, pumping loads of hormones into the system. The body releases adrenaline, and blood pressure and heart rate increase. These are all useful if you're dodging a dinosaur out by the watering hole but a little excessive if you're just getting jostled on a city sidewalk.

The fight-or-flight reflex is also kicked off by stress, which probably edges out hostility as the most pervasive of all the modern ills. "I am convinced that stress is a primary cause or aggravating factor in many conditions that bring patients to doctors," writes Andrew Weil, M.D., director of the Program in Integrative Medicine at the University of Arizona College of Medicine in Tucson and author of several books, including *Spontaneous Healing*. Researchers suspect that stress reduces the supply of oxygen to the heart while simultaneously increasing demand for it. People who react strongly to stress have been shown to be three times more likely to have a heart attack or need heart surgery than those who don't.

The Mind-Body Upside

Although a lot of the mind-body research conducted so far has focused on the harmful potential of negative emotions, there's plenty of evidence showing that our feelings can be our allies, too. One of the groundbreaking mind-body studies conducted at Stanford University found that being in a support group helped cancer patients stay in remission and, therefore, live longer.

The message of this study is clear: There are ways that the mind's self-healing potential can be marshaled to overcome less-than-optimal conditions. One of the leaders in showing how we can do just that is Herbert Benson, M.D., associate professor of medicine at Harvard Medical School and president of the Mind/Body Medical Institute at New England Deaconess Hospital in Boston. Dr. Benson developed the "relaxation response," a simple four-step meditation technique that enables patients to lower their blood pressures, their heart rates, their rates of breathing, and their muscle tension. He calls the calming effect of the relaxation response the opposite effect of the fight-or-flight response and says that it can alter the way the body reacts to stress after the exercise itself has been completed.

And this isn't the only such method to have been developed. Techniques as various as prayer, yoga, tai chi, and even knitting can elicit the same response. So can exercise.

Another key to marshaling the body's self-healing resources is attitude. Research has shown that the way we interpret and react to life's trials can determine how they affect our immune systems. One study conducted at the University of Chicago observed 200 telecommunications executives as their company went through a downsizing. Those who survived the transition with their good health intact tended to see change as an opportunity for growth rather than as a threat. They also had strong networks of social support and a deep sense of commitment to their jobs and to their families. Executives who possessed these qualities of "psychological hardiness" had less than a 33 percent chance of contracting a severe illness during or soon after the downsizing process, while executives who didn't possess them had a probability of severe illness that was higher than 9 chances in 10.

The Next Step

While great progress has been made in uncovering the mysteries of the mind-body connection, much more remains to be learned. We don't understand, for example, exactly how emotions predispose us for disease. Nor are we close to fathoming how far the mind-body connection can take us.

Another mystery is the degree to which people may be able to influence health through prayer. Prayer and meditation can definitely have an impact on physiology. Dr. Benson reports that 25 percent of his patients report feeling "more spiritual" after practicing the relaxation response (regardless of whether the focus of their exercise was of a religious nature).

A 1994 study on the impact of religious views on health showed not only that religious people tend to be healthier on average than the population as a whole (in part because they are less likely to smoke cigarettes or consume alcohol) but also that they have less anxiety, less depression, and less hostility. They also live longer.

The $64,000 question is whether such benefits are the result solely of their faith and their lifestyle or whether religious people are receiving outside help, either from other religious people who pray for them or from some other source. These are not the kinds of phenomena that scientists feel comfortable investigating, but Dr. Pert says that the implications of mind-body research keep pointing inexorably in that direction. "It's pretty esoteric stuff," she says, "but emotions seem to be able to leap from one person to another. That gets into some very mysterious areas that, for want of a better word, we have to call spiritual. We may not have the physics down yet, but there may well be a scientific basis for spirituality."

Rethinking the Placebo Effect

Placebo is Latin for "I will please," and it's used to describe the fact that people often respond to medical treatment because they *think* they'll get better, not because of the treatment's physiological effects. Researchers habitually test new drugs by giving the real drug to one group of test subjects and sugar pills—placebos—to another group. (The subjects don't know which pills they receive.) If the drug doesn't perform better than the placebo, it's a flop.

The placebo effect is thought to derive from a combination of several different powers of suggestion, chief among them the patient's belief in the skills of his doctor, the patient's belief in the effectiveness of a particular treatment (whether it be a drug, surgery, a massage, or a prayer), and the doctor's belief in the power of his treatment. Whatever the reasons, no one doubts that the placebo effect works. The results are often anything but imaginary. Patients have been known to develop skin rashes when they took placebos, for example. The rashes went away as soon as the "medication" was stopped, returning when the placebo was resumed.

Recognizing the powerful influence of the mind-body connection, the holistic practitioner embraces the placebo effect as an important ally in the service of his main goal: helping patients feel better. "Who cares whether it's placebo?" asks Dr. Bruce Pomeranz of the University of Toronto Medical School. "If it works, that's all that matters. And if it works with fewer side effects than prescription drugs or surgery, that's even better."

Herbal Origins

Where Natural Remedies Come From

Wanna take a trip around the world?

Go to your nearest health food store and visit the herb section. What you'll see there is a rich and heady mixture of plants from different cultures and different healing traditions. They may look innocuous enough in their bottles and packages, but considering where they've come from, it's as if you've walked into a crowded marketplace in some exotic foreign land, a place where the colors are bright, the smells intoxicating, and the customs mysterious. Pause at any of the market's stalls, and you'll hear some wonderful stories. To illustrate our point, we'll talk here about the far-flung origins of some of the most common and most effective herbs you'll come across in your perusing.

Consider St.-John's-wort, for example. Thanks to copious media coverage, most Americans are now aware that St.-John's-wort works as an organic antidepressant. This was not exactly news to people who have used the plant they called the Devil's Scourge for thousands of years to ward off evil spirits.

St.-John's-wort grows wild in much of northern Europe. Colonists brought it to America, and soon it grew wild here, too. It became so prevalent, in fact, that ranchers considered it a noxious weed and tried to stamp it out. (Cattle can develop a hypersensitivity to sunlight when they eat St.-John's-wort, as can humans. It may be this property that makes it an effective treatment for de-

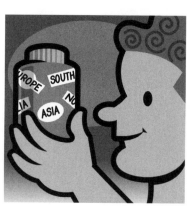

pression for people who live in cloudy, gloomy climates, since it helps the skin absorb more efficiently what sunlight there is.)

Most of the St.-John's-wort that you buy in stores has for years been gathered mainly from the wild (the term that herbalists use for this is *wildcrafting*). But now, the demand has grown so great that it's being cultivated, frantically, by farmers. "People can't grow enough of it," says Cascade Anderson Geller, an herbal educator and consultant in Portland, Oregon.

The Native American Contribution

North America has given medicinal herbs to the world as well as received them. Goldenseal is a good example. A small, fragile plant that grows in shady woodlands, it was used by Cherokees and Iroquois as a treatment for everything from cancer to diarrhea. Eventually, immigrants to North America caught on, and goldenseal is now one of the best-selling herbal remedies around, used as an ingredient in more than 500 products, especially in Germany and France. That popularity presents a problem since goldenseal is not a plant that readily lends itself to cultivation, and wild sources are rapidly being cleaned out. As a result, goldenseal is now listed as an endangered species in at least a half-dozen states; herbalists worry that it may become extinct.

Echinacea, another herbal remedy used by Native Americans, may be even more popular than goldenseal: Surveys have consistently listed it as the best-selling herbal supplement in health food stores. Wild supplies are disappearing, but unlike goldenseal, some varieties of echinacea can be easily cultivated for sale. And they are, at a tremendous rate.

From the Tropics

For variety of plants and potential medicines, nothing beats tropical rain forests. One reason that rain forests are such rich sources of herbal medicines is the sheer stress of survival that the plants endure. Any given plant in the jungle competes for life with a host of insect predators. Plants protect themselves by producing chemicals that are toxic to insects, thereby deterring predation. These same chemical weapons may have medicinal effects when ingested by humans.

Quinine is a case in point. It's derived from the bark of the cinchona tree and has an extremely bitter taste, which makes it an unpalatable lunch for would-be predators. Cinchona bark was known as a cure for malaria as far back as the Incas.

And that's just one of many important drugs that have emerged from tropical jungles. Whether the miracle drugs of tomorrow will have the opportunity to emerge is another question. Although drug companies and botanists are actively collecting and analyzing plants in various habitats around the world, environmental destruction of those habitats is a growing concern. "Every day, we lose another 2,500 acres of natural habitat in the United States to development," says Richard Liebmann, N.D., a naturopathic physician and executive director of United Plant Savers, an organization based in East Barre, Vermont, that is dedicated to preserving native American medicinal plants. Of the 150 or so medicinal plants sold in this country, Dr. Liebmann adds, nearly a third are in some danger of being wiped out.

Brainy and Resilient

Some medicinal plants, thankfully, seem to have come to terms with civilization more

Truth in Labeling

When scientists venture into remote regions to learn from the natives which plants have healing powers, they must be aware not only of natural predators, but of their own naïveté.

In his book *Tales of a Shaman's Apprentice*, ethnobotanist Mark J. Plotkin, Ph.D., reports that researchers exploring South American jungles dutifully took down and published a long name for a certain plant. When translated into English, the name turned out to mean "I don't know this one, so I'll have to ask my uncle." Another researcher listed the common name of a plant thought to cure constipation as *kakabrokoe*. Roughly translated, *kakabrokoe* means "poop in your pants."

readily than others. The ginkgo tree is an example. One of the oldest living tree species on Earth, ginkgo fossils have been uncovered that are 280 million years old, reports ethnobotanist Dr. Mark J. Plotkin in his book *Tales of a Shaman's Apprentice*. Long extinct in the wild, the ginkgo survived and flourished in the temples of China and Japan. From there, it has spread around the world. The ginkgo seems impervious to both predators and pollution, among other environmental threats. It is said that the blackened remains of a ginkgo growing near ground zero in Hiroshima sprouted leaves a few months after the city was leveled.

Ginkgo's ability to stimulate blood flow to the brain has made it a popular supplement in Europe for decades. More recently, it began catching on in a big way in the United States. Suppliers are struggling to keep up with demand—so much so that the ginkgo leaves you buy in your health food store tomorrow may have been stripped by unscrupulous natural-supplement suppliers, under cover of darkness, from a tree growing on your block last year.

From the East

Two Ancient Systems of Healing

In the Raymond Chandler novel *Farewell, My Lovely,* the quintessential hard-boiled Los Angeles private eye, Philip Marlowe, goes up against a "psychic consultant" who cultivates a sense of exotic mystery of vaguely Eastern origins.

At their first meeting, Marlowe awaits the psychic in a darkened, velvet-draped room lit only by a milk-white globe on a black stand. The psychic enters and tries to stare Marlowe down with deep, black pitiless eyes.

"Please do not fidget," the psychic says. "It breaks the waves, disturbs my concentration."

"It makes the ice melt, the butter run, and the cat squawk," Marlowe replies.

Good old Marlowe wasn't buying that mumbo jumbo for a second, and most of us like to think that we wouldn't either. You won't find any psychic charlatans in this book, but you will discover that a lot of alternative therapies come from Eastern cultures, and they work. In fact, they've been working for thousands of years.

The sheer length of time that Asian and Indian civilizations have been around means that they've preserved connections to natural, spiritually oriented healing techniques that Westerners have abandoned or never had. When you've been hacking away at something for 3,000 years or more, you tend to get a certain groove going.

The two ancient systems of healing that have the greatest influence on alternative healing in the United States today are Traditional Chinese Medicine and the Indian practice of

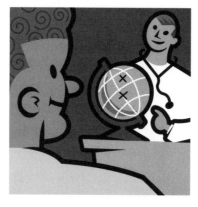

Ayurveda. Both are very old, and both have much in common, although they also have many differences. Here's an overview of each.

Traditional Chinese Medicine

The healing philosophies that evolved in China over thousands of years—archaeologists have uncovered acupuncture needles dating back to 1000 B.C.—are holistic in the truest sense of the word. All of creation is seen to be interconnected and in relationship. The best symbol of that interrelationship is the yin/yang sign, which represents the basic forces of the cosmos in constant interaction with one another. Good health results from a proper balance of those forces. An imbalance leads to illness, and the goal of medicine is to correct that imbalance.

This emphasis on remaining in harmony with nature means that Chinese medicine is more oriented than Western medicine toward staying healthy in the first place, rather than on fixing a disease once it occurs. The Chinese predilection toward harmony and balance also means that their physicians take it for granted that a person's emotional and physical environment will have a profound impact on his physical well-being. Similarly, the graceful movements of Chinese exercise disciplines such as chi kung and tai chi are methods of enhancing the flow of energy through the body, as are the Indian techniques of yoga. Meditation, a key adjunct to Traditional Chinese Medicine, serves the same purpose.

The two basic treatment methods in Chinese medicine are acupuncture and herbs.

Acupuncture. This system of healing is based on the idea that there are 12 main channels (meridians) running through the body, much like the circulatory system, through which the life force (chi) flows. Each of these meridians is lined with specific points that serve as portals into this river of chi. When a needle is inserted at one of those points, or when one of those points is massaged by hand (as in acupressure), blockages that hinder the proper flow of energy through the body can be released. Acupuncture needles penetrate just below the surface of the skin, and they're very thin, so the treatment isn't painful. It generally doesn't draw blood, although sterilized and disposable needles should be used. Sometimes, heat or electrical stimulation is applied through the needles for additional effect.

To Western minds, how a needle inserted in one part of your body can relieve pain somewhere else seems hard to comprehend. But in 1997, a panel convened by the National Institutes of Health (NIH) concluded that acupuncture can be considered an effective treatment for a number of conditions, including nausea following surgery and chemotherapy, pain following dental surgery, lower-back pain, and tennis elbow. The NIH also cited studies that suggested that acupuncture might be helpful in treating a long list of additional conditions, among them postoperative pain, addiction, stroke rehabilitation, carpal tunnel syndrome, arthritis, and headache. The NIH's findings were seen as a breakthrough in acceptance by the medical establishment, but acupuncturists still consider them very conservative. By comparison, the World Health Organization lists more than 40 conditions for which acupuncture treatments may be useful.

Chinese herbal medicine. As strange as acupuncture may seem, there are elements to Chinese herbal medicine that may seem a little stranger. A few herbal remedies in the Chinese tradition consist of single herbs—ginseng and ginkgo are probably the best-known—but

The Ever-Shifting Balance

There's a great irony to all the attention we Westerners are paying these days to the healing practices of the East. In the East, there's an equal attraction to the healing practices of the West. Another case of the grass always being greener? At least one doctor who's familiar with both sides of the world believes that something more cosmic is at work.

The fact that both East and West seem at this point to be turning toward one another is entirely consistent with the characteristics represented by the yin/yang symbol, suggests Dr. M. Kyu Chung of Cooper Health Systems.

Western medicine is very "yang" in nature, Dr. Chung believes, because it tends to be aggressive and direct, whereas Eastern medicine is "yin" because its character tends to be more indirect and nurturing. In each half of that symbol, there is a dot of the opposite color. Those dots represent the tendency of both yin and yang to move in each other's direction. "Over the course of time," Dr. Chung says, "the yin will become yang, and the yang will become yin."

From that perspective, by seeking out each other's healing practices, both East and West are behaving exactly as they should be.

most are complicated mixtures designed specifically for individual patients. A typical prescription could contain a dozen ingredients or more. Although animal parts are rarely used in herbal medicine today, items such as cicada husks and silkworms can be part of a recipe. This is not the kind of product you're likely to see on the shelves of your local drugstore anytime soon, but don't let the oddities throw you off. Chinese herbal remedies seem to work. "Chinese herbs can be valuable for treating most simple or chronic problems, anything that doesn't need dramatic chemical or surgical intervention," says Ted Kaptchuk, a doctor of Oriental medicine, herbalist, and acupuncturist in Cambridge, Massachusetts, and author of *Web That Has No Weaver*, a book about Chinese medicine.

Ayurveda

India's Ayurveda ("science of life") is rooted in the ancient religious texts of Hinduism, which scholars say are more than 5,000 years old. The idea of staying in balance with the forces of nature is as intrinsic to Ayurveda as it is to Traditional Chinese Medicine. So is the concept of a central life force, which the Indians call *prana*. Ayurveda is also deeply holistic in the sense that the body is seen as an expression of divine intelligence. Ill health results from falling out of tune with that divine intelligence, which is seen as a case of "mistaken intellect."

The Ayurvedic system sees *prana* as being expressed in each individual through his *dosha*, an inborn personality and physical type. There are three types of *dosha*: *kapha*, *pitta*, and *vata*. The *doshas* are Ayurveda's equivalent to the yin/yang sign in that they are symbolic descriptions of cosmic forces in action and in interaction. Every individual has a different balance of *doshas*, determined at the moment of conception. Good health is the result of the *doshas* being in proper balance. Specific types of imbalance will lead to particular types of illness.

Like their counterparts in Chinese medicine, Ayurvedic practitioners tend to spend a lot of time examining their patients. That's because in both systems, diagnosis is as much an art as a science, with a heavy emphasis on observation. The

---

Dosha Dictionary

Ayurveda is a lot easier to understand once you know which qualities in a person and which body functions are associated with each of the three *doshas* (Ayurvedic categories). See which category you fall into.

Kapha: Water and earth; associated with the body's lubricating fluids. Caring, sensuous, centered, compassionate, good-humored, faithful, patient, down-to-earth, supportive. Kapha personalities tend to be steady and reliable, sometimes to a fault.

Pitta: Fire; involved with digestion, maintenance of body temperature, and assimilation of mental experiences. Ambition, passion, determination, confidence, enthusiasm for knowledge, happiness, intelligence. A pitta constitution tends to be alert and focused.

Vata: Air; involved with alertness and movement (circulation, reflexes, heartbeat, and so on). Creativity, enthusiasm, generosity, exuberance. Vata personalities are likely to be artistic and resourceful; actual execution of these ideas can be another matter.

---

texture of the hair, the color and condition of the eyes and skin, the smell of the body and of the breath, and, most of all, the rhythm and intensity of the pulse are all taken into account. Both systems also consider home and work environments to be powerful influences on physical well-being.

Ayurvedic treatments emphasize a healthy diet, heavy on fresh vegetables, fruits, and grains. Other components of a standard course of treatment might include courses in yoga and meditation as well as counseling on work and sleep habits. Herbs might be prescribed, either as additions to the diet (cumin and ginger are two of the better-known herbs in the Ayurvedic kitchen) or, in more serious cases, as medicinal preparations in a wide variety of forms.

Other Healing Philosophies

Helping the Body Heal Itself

Talk to some alternative medicine practitioners long enough, and it's easy to get the impression that when it comes to healing, man may have stopped making sense about 100 years ago, and that any ideas more recent than that are downright dangerous to your health.

In truth, two of the mainstays of the alternative healing movement are neither ancient nor completely modern. One, naturopathy, originated near the turn of the twentieth century, although it draws on ideas about health that date back much further than that, blending them with modern understandings of anatomy, physiology, biochemistry, and nutrition. The other, homeopathy, is 200 years old. It, too, connects to ideas from the more-distant past, although it has also developed some pretty unique concepts of its own.

Naturopathy and homeopathy share a fundamental belief that the body is its own best healer, and that it is the physician's job to assist that self-healing process. In that pursuit, naturopathic doctors take a broad-based approach. They are the general practitioners of natural healing, orchestra conductors who can bring a whole symphony of holistic techniques to bear on a given problem—or on staying healthy so that problems don't develop in the first place. One of the main techniques that naturopaths use is homeopathy, which shares many of natur-

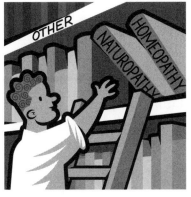

opathy's basic principles. Here's an overview of both disciplines.

Naturopathy

Naturopathy came to the United States at the turn of the twentieth century. It's an offshoot of a European approach to healing called the Nature Cure, which advocated natural foods, pure water, fresh air, sunshine, exercise, and hydrotherapy (steam baths and the like) as the route to good health.

The naturopaths' broad range of diagnostic and treatment skills are based on a classic holistic philosophy. They believe that a range of internal and external influences can contribute to the onset of any illness and that taking all those various influences into account is important in achieving both an immediate cure and ongoing health. Naturopaths also consider teaching their patients the fundamentals of healthful living to be one of their chief responsibilities. The original root of the word *doctor*, they are fond of pointing out, means "teacher."

Virtually any naturopathic practice includes a strong emphasis on diet, nutrition (the use of vitamins, minerals, and other supplements), and herbal remedies. Most naturopaths also have training in such physical therapies as spinal manipulation, hydrotherapy, and massage and will be familiar with at least the basics of homeopathy, acupuncture, and counseling. A given practice will typically concentrate on a few of these disciplines, so it's important to check to see that the therapeutic menu of any naturopath you visit covers the specific areas you want to address.

Naturopaths consider themselves primary care physicians: When you're sick, they want you to come to them first. It's their job, as they see it, to assess your condition, decide on appropriate treatments, and (when necessary) make a referral to another doctor. If a patient needs his appendix removed or his heart repaired, he'll be turned over to a conventional M.D. But the naturopaths' emphasis on holistic treatment means that they try to avoid automatically referring patients out to a long line of specialists who each focus on one narrow part of the body.

"The idea is more to look at the whole person and see how all his various health problems might be related," says Tim Birdsall, N.D., a naturopathic physician in Sandpoint, Idaho; vice president of the American Association of Naturopathic Physicians in Seattle; and editor-in-chief of *Alternative Medicine Review.* In Dr. Birdsall's practice, about 10 percent of the patients at some time have problems that need treatment or diagnosis by other doctors.

As their name implies, naturopaths believe strongly in the healing power of nature, and as a result, they'll try to find the least invasive, least pharmaceutical route to wellness that is available.

Another key element of their philosophy is that the symptoms of a given disease are evidence of the body trying to heal itself. For that reason, naturopaths don't consider it their job to get rid of symptoms; rather, the goal is to try to understand the underlying causes toward which the symptoms point. Frequent colds, for example, might point to a more systemic weakness in the immune system or to an allergy, while chronic headaches might suggest a problem with stress or low blood sugar. Symptom stoppers like aspirin or cough syrup can be helpful now and then, but not if they are used consistently to mask what is really going on.

"Every disease has a beginning, a middle, and an end," says Thomas Kruzel, N.D., a naturopathic physician in Portland, Oregon, and former president of the American Association of Naturopathic Physicians. "When the healing process is suppressed, healing doesn't get a chance to reach completion."

Homeopathy

To its critics—and there are many—homeopathy is another name for snake oil. To its advocates—and there are many of those, too—it's a powerful yet gentle system of healing that stimulates the body's inherent ability to cure itself. How exactly this occurs even they don't pretend to understand.

Homeopathy began in the late eighteenth century when a well-educated German physician named Samuel Hahnemann explored what would become known as the law of similars. Simply put, the idea is that certain substances create specific physical symptoms when taken by healthy people. If sick people who exhibit those same physical symptoms take small doses of those same substances, the thinking goes, their natural defense mechanisms will be stimulated, and they will be cured.

Dr. Hahnemann tested various substances on healthy people and meticulously documented the symptoms they provoked. Today, there are more than 1,300 homeopathic remedies that are made from plant, mineral, or animal sources. The list includes more than a few things you wouldn't think would be all that healthy to consume, including belladonna, arsenic, crushed bees, and snake venom.

Dr. Hahnemann also discovered the principle of potentizing. Homeopathic remedies are prepared by diluting the active ingredient in water or alcohol, shaking it, and diluting it again. In many cases, these dilutions are repeated so often that no trace—not a single molecule—of the active ingredient remains. No matter; the principle of potentizing holds that the therapeutic effect of the remedy actually increases the more it is diluted.

No explanation for this curious phenomenon has been discovered either, although homeopaths are optimistic that science will one day provide an answer. In the meantime, the one point skeptics and true believers seem to agree on is that, regardless of whether homeopathic remedies do any good, the principle of potentizing virtually guarantees that they won't do any harm.

The basic idea of the law of similars was known and practiced by the ancient Greeks. Today, conventional immunization stimulates the body's immune system to produce antibodies in order to kill an artificially introduced infection. The difference is that scientists can measure the presence of those antibodies in the bloodstream of someone who has had a vaccination, whereas no such physiological result can be discerned when homeopathic remedies are administered. All that is known is that people seem to get better. The credit is given, once more, to the body's own powerful ability to heal itself. But how that occurs is a mystery.

Research illustrating homeopathy's effectiveness is increasing. A study by the Centre for Complementary Medicine Research in Munich, Germany, showed that homeopathic remedies were 66 percent more effective than a placebo was. As the research continues, so does the steady stream of satisfied patients leaving their homeopath's office. "I'm a clinician, not a research scientist," says Stephen Messer, N.D., a diplomate of the Homeopathic Academy of Naturopathic Physicians and a naturopathic and homeopathic physician in private practice in Eugene, Oregon. "This stuff works. I can't tell you that I help everybody who comes to see me, but I help a lot of people whom nobody else could help, and that's very rewarding."

In answer to the skeptics' charge that homeopathy works because patients and doctors believe it works— also known as the placebo effect—homeopaths say that they've seen their remedies cure countless infants and animals as well as adults. They also point to the widespread use of homeopathy around the world. As many as 70 percent of physicians in France consider homeopathy effective, for example, while 42

Homeopathy's Greatest Hits

Here are the five most popular over-the-counter homeopathic remedies and what they're good for, according to Michael Traub, N.D., a diplomate of the Homeopathic Academy of Naturopathic Physicians, chief of the scientific affairs department of the American Association of Naturopathic Physicians in Seattle, and a naturopathic and homeopathic physician in Kailua Kona, Hawaii.

Arnica montana: Used for bruises, muscle strains, and sprains, this remedy is also useful before and after surgery to reduce trauma.

Pulsatilla: This remedy is used for colds, flu, ear and eye infections, hay fever, and prostate infections.

Nux vomica: This remedy is good for digestion problems resulting from too much food or alcohol. Also helpful for colds, flu, insomnia (specifically, for insomnia "due to thoughts about work or how to accomplish tasks," Dr. Traub says), hemorrhoids, constipation, hay fever, and prostate infections.

Arsenicum album: Made from arsenic, this remedy is good for heartburn, stomachache, food poisoning, diarrhea, colds, flu, cough, sore throat, insomnia (due to "general anxiety"), and hay fever.

Rhus toxicodendron: Made from poison ivy, this remedy helps with colds, flu, sore throats, laryngitis (due to "overuse of the voice"), muscle strains and stiffness (resulting from accidents), arthritis, bursitis, tendinitis, and poison oak.

percent of physicians in Britain referred patients to homeopathic doctors, according to Dana Ullman, founder of Homeopathic Educational Services in Berkeley, California, and author of *The Consumer's Guide to Homeopathy*. In Germany, more than $400 million worth of homeopathic remedies are sold each year, Ullman reports, and 85 percent of those sales represent prescriptions from physicians.

What does homeopathy cure, if indeed it cures? Just about anything, from colds, flu, bruises, and jet lag to asthma, depression, and swollen prostate glands. Serious health problems should be left for a conventional medical doctor to diagnose and treat, but a wide range of lesser ailments can be alleviated, homeopaths say, by remedies that are available in health food stores and in national retail chains such as Kmart, Walgreens, and CVS. The difference between buying homeopathic remedies over the counter and getting them from a homeopath is the difference between attacking your illness with a shotgun and a rifle, says Michael Carlston, M.D., assistant clinical professor in the department of family and community medicine at the University of California, San Francisco, School of Medicine and a homeopathic physician in Santa Rosa, California. The over-the-counter varieties tend to be remedies that address a broad range of health problems—often several different remedies are combined—which means that they won't necessarily address the systemic problems that underlie the current illness.

Homeopaths take great pride in pinpointing, exactly, each patient's specific problem. The number of symptoms listed in the "provings" (tests of substances on healthy people and the reactions they provoked) for

Trolling for Therapies

Virtually every alternative therapy has a national organization that can give you more information on its practices and practitioners. Here's a list of the major ones.

Acupuncture and Traditional Chinese Medicine
American Academy of Medical Acupuncture (AAMA)
5820 Wilshire Boulevard, Suite 500
Los Angeles, CA 90036-4500

National Commission for the Certification
   of Acupuncture and Oriental Medicine
11 Canal Center Plaza, Suite 300
Alexandria, VA 22314-1595

Biofeedback
Association for Applied Psychophysiology and
   Biofeedback
10200 West 44th Avenue, Suite 304
Wheat Ridge, CO 80033-2840

Cognitive Therapy
Beck Institute for Cognitive Therapy and Research
1 Belmont Avenue, Suite 700
Bala Cynwyd, PA 19004-1610

Herbal Therapy
Herb Research Foundation
1007 Pearl Street, Suite 200
Boulder, CO 80302-5124

Homeopathy
National Center for Homeopathy
801 North Fairfax Street, Suite 306
Alexandria, VA 22314-1757

many of the homeopathic remedies is remarkable, as is their precision. That's why if you visit a homeopath's office with a chronic condition, you'll be grilled on everything from the color and consistency of the mucus you're spitting up to the times you break out in a sweat, the temperature of the liquids you're drinking, and the sorts of foods you crave. You're also likely to be

Homeopathic Educational Services
2124 Kittredge Street
Berkeley, CA 94704-1436

Hydrotherapy
Uchee Pines Institute
30 Uchee Pines Road, Suite 75
Seale, AL 36875-5702

Imagery
Academy for Guided Imagery
P. O. Box 2070
Mill Valley, CA 94942-2070

Massage
American Massage Therapy Association
820 Davis Street, Suite 100
Evanston, IL 60201-4464

Music Therapy
American Music Therapy Association
8455 Colesville Road, Suite 1000
Silver Spring, MD 20910-3392

Naturopathic Medicine
American Association of Naturopathic
    Physicians
601 Valley Street, Suite 105
Seattle, WA 98109-4229

Yoga
American Yoga Association
513 South Orange Avenue, Suite 1
Sarasota, FL 34236-7598

goes to his reference books and matches it as closely as possible with the homeopathic remedy that produced the same set of symptoms in the provings. It is this attention to detail that homeopaths say distinguishes their prescriptions from the "one diagnosis fits all" approach of conventional medicine.

Homeopathic remedies come in different concentrations and are marked with a number and either an "X," for the decimal scale, which means that potencies are diluted 10 times each time that they are shaken, or a "C," for the centesimal scale, which means that potencies are diluted 100 times each time that they are shaken. The greater the number, the more powerful the substance will be, yet the more dilute it is, according to proponents of homeopathy.

Homeopaths also share with naturopaths the conviction that symptoms are signs of the body's natural healing process. Dr. Kruzel, who uses homeopathy as a central part of his naturopathy practice, recalls one patient, a 38-year-old man, who came to him with a testicular infection. It turned out that a few weeks earlier, he had developed a rash on the end of his penis, which he had attempted to get rid of with a topical cortisone cream. The rash had indeed cleared up, Dr. Kruzel says—or appeared to. In truth, what happened is that the cortisone cream only drove the infection deeper into the man's body, and the testicular infection was the result. When Dr. Kruzel treated the testicular infection with a homeopathic remedy, he was not surprised to see the original penile rash return. "He was healing," Dr. Kruzel says, "in reverse order." A second homeopathic remedy cleared up the rash, and the man was cured.

asked about your sex life, bowel habits, and moods. "Practically all of my patients really appreciate the opportunity to discuss their health without interruption," says Nicholas Nossaman, M.D., a family medicine and homeopathic physician in private practice in Denver.

Once a comprehensive picture of characteristics has been assembled, the homeopath

Alternative Terminology

Who Does What?

When in doubt, make a chart.

That's our motto. The idea here is to provide you with two types of overview: one of each type of therapy, the other of the alternative landscape as a whole—the forest and the trees, if you will.

The "trees" perspective may be especially useful as a reference when you're consulting the power programs we've laid out in Part Three, or the healing regimens for specific health problems in Part Four. Refer back to the chart for a quick reminder of the basics for a given modality. Scanning through the chart before you dive into the rest of the book will give you a good sense of the territory—the forest—we're going to cover.

Note that the chart reveals quite clearly the major patterns that crop up repeatedly in the various alternative therapies. These include:

Age. Alternative healing methods tend to be old, thousands of years old in several cases.

Lack of research. The antiquity of these methods means that many of them originated long before the scientific method did. Hence, they often have not been subjected to the kinds of research studies that conventional medicine, which developed much later, views as a pre-

Approach	What It Is	How It Works	Where It Came From
Acupressure	This therapy uses your hands and fingers to put pressure on strategic points of the body for relieving pain, reducing symptoms of illness, and promoting health.	Health is obtained by maintaining a balance of vital energy (*chi*); an imbalance signifies disease. Acupressure relieves symptoms of illness by triggering production of neurochemicals, which ferry information between your brain and body.	It originated in China more than 2,500 years ago.
Acupuncture	Insertion of needles at strategic points in the body relieves pain, treats illness, and promotes health.	Acupuncture may relieve symptoms of illness by triggering production of neurochemicals, which ferry information between your brain and body.	It has been used in China as one component of Traditional Chinese Medicine, which dates back some 2,500 years.
Ayurveda	This holistic method combines medicinal and preventive remedies with diet, yoga, and meditation.	The cornerstone to diagnosis and treatment is through determination of your *dosha* (a physical/mental/spiritual categorization). Emphasis is placed on specific diets to maintain balanced *doshas*.	In India, the principles of Ayurveda were codified in the religious texts of Hinduism more than 5,000 years ago.

requisite for legitimacy. Whether that makes a given therapy less reliable depends upon whom you talk to and your own biases. In any event, research scientists are conducting a steadily growing number of studies on various alternative methods.

Holism. Alternative treatments tend to involve the whole person rather than an isolated organ or specific symptom. The fact that mind, body, and spirit affect one another is generally accepted as a basic assumption. Holism also means that alternative practitioners typically place a higher priority on promotion of overall health and the prevention of illness than conventional doctors do.

Exoticism. The chart demonstrates why some people consider *alternative* a euphemism for *weird*. Again, age has a lot to do with that: Many of these practices emerged from ancient civ-

ilizations that occupied a psychic universe vastly different from our own. Even some of the newer modalities, such as homeopathy or naturopathy, draw on wisdom that extends back centuries.

The exoticism of the alternative world is one of its greatest attractions or one of its most glaring defects, depending on your point of view. Then there are those who don't really care about the trappings; they're only interested in what works. There's plenty of that here, too.

Professionalism. As you review the chart, you'll note that we have a category, "Who Does It," listing the professional designations of accredited practitioners in each healing discipline. But also bear in mind that M.D.'s and Ph.D.'s who have training or experience in the outlined modes of healing might also be appropriate to consult.

Who Does It*	What It's Good For	Acceptance	Factoid
An O.M.D., L.Ac., or L.M.T. performs acupressure. Membership in the American Oriental Bodywork Therapy Association is helpful.	It alleviates and prevents stress-related aches and pains, allergies, nausea, sinus problems, and constipation. It also helps to heal sports injuries and lessen anxiety, depression, insomnia, and a range of other problems.	Millions of Chinese people use it, and it is embraced by many American physicians and health professionals as a powerful method for pain relief and disease treatment.	You've already used acupressure if you've ever rubbed your temples when your head hurt or held your stomach when you've had a stomachache.
Practitioners have an O.M.D., L.Ac., or certification from the National Commission for the Certification of Acupuncture and Oriental Medicine in Washington, D.C.	It is especially renowned for helping with nausea, vomiting, and pain relief.	The National Institutes of Health stated that acupuncture is an effective treatment for certain conditions and recommends expansion of its use in conventional medicine.	Despite its long history, acupuncture was largely unknown in the United States until 1971, when former President Richard Nixon reestablished ties with China.
Look for an N.D. or O.M.D. with training in Ayurveda; a member of the Council of Maharishi Ayur-Veda Physicians; or an individual with a B.A.M.S., a degree from India that is roughly equivalent to a Western M.D.	Ayurveda treats all ailments by treating the whole person and not just the person's health problems.	Ayurveda is widely practiced in India and elsewhere. Maharishi Ayur-Veda is one of the two types of Ayurvedic medicine practiced in the United States.	*Ayurveda* is Sanskrit for "the science of life."

(*continued*)

Approach	What It Is	How It Works	Where It Came From
Biofeedback	This treatment helps you learn to control some of the body's vital functions that affect your health.	Your blood pressure, temperature, muscle tension, heartbeat, or brain waves are monitored and turned into easy-to-interpret sounds or images in an effort to teach you how to control them.	Medical science first tuned in to biofeedback in the 1960s.
Cognitive Therapy	This short-term therapy focuses on getting you to change your behavior and your general outlook, focusing on the present and not the past.	Among other tactics, you'll learn how your thoughts influence your emotions and behavior, and how to apply new thinking to your daily life.	It was developed by psychologist Aaron T. Beck, M.D., in the 1960s.
Herbal Therapy	This method uses plants to treat disease and maintain good health.	The therapeutic effects of a plant result from the combined action of the many compounds within the plant working together.	Since the dawn of humanity, herbal remedies have existed. But scientific study of herbs didn't begin until the eighteenth century.
Homeopathy	This modality is based on the principle that "like cures like." Medical conditions are treated by administering a minute dose of a remedy that would, in larger doses, produce the medical condition's symptoms.	Unlike conventional medicine, homeopathy doesn't treat symptoms but treats whatever is disturbing your system and creating those symptoms.	This remedy was developed about 200 years ago by Samuel Hahnemann, a German physician.
Hydrotherapy	Different temperatures of water are applied in various ways and methods to ease a host of complaints.	Through baths, saunas, whirlpools, body wraps, or compresses, hydrotherapy is thought to increase circulation and speed healing.	As a healing discipline, it was officially born in the early 1800s when a German farmer used cold compresses to heal his broken ribs.
Imagery and Visualization	This technique uses thoughts to control illness, deal with pain, or reach goals.	The relaxation response that visualization and imagery create counterbalances stress and the symptoms that stress causes.	This therapy was used by the ancient Egyptians and by American Indian tribes thousands of years ago.

Who Does It*	What It's Good For	Acceptance	Factoid
One with a B.C.I.A.-C. provides this therapy.	Biofeedback is noted for its ability to help with headaches, circulation problems, stroke rehabilitation, alcoholism, and post-traumatic stress syndrome.	It is used by conventional M.D.'s, psychologists, and psychiatrists to help relieve stress-related complaints and other health conditions.	A study found that Vietnam veterans who used biofeedback were able to reduce their intake of psychiatric medications.
See a mental health professional with a background in cognitive therapy. For severe disorders, consult a psychologist (Ph.D.) or psychiatrist (M.D.).	Cognitive therapy can relieve a long list of emotionally related problems, including anxiety, depression, high blood pressure, marital difficulties, and weight problems.	Approximately 3,000 practitioners are trained in cognitive therapy in the United States.	A study at the University of California, Los Angeles, indicated that cognitive therapy may actually alter the chemistry of the brain.
Visit a Traditional Chinese Medicine doctor (such as an O.M.D.), licensed N.D., or a professional member of the A.H.G.	It's good for a variety of ailments, from fighting viral and bacterial infection to reducing risk of coronary artery disease.	Medical schools such as Harvard and Cornell have programs that provide some level of herbal instruction.	The dandelions growing in your backyard are herbal remedies (if you don't use pesticides) that help fight disease.
Some M.D.'s and D.O.'s are board-certified and add D.Ht. to their credentials. Certified N.D.'s use D.H.A.N.P. Other practitioners use C.C.H.	Studies in Europe have shown positive results for conditions such as diarrhea and hay fever.	Homeopathy use is growing in the United States and is widely practiced in Europe, Latin America, and Asia.	About 40 percent of British, French, and Dutch doctors use homeopathy, and 20 percent of German doctors do.
Go to a licensed N.D. or someone who has completed course study in hydrotherapy from a school or professional association.	It's good for treating nasal congestion, stress, and insomnia.	It is a component of naturopathy used regularly by naturopathic doctors, among others.	Hydrotherapy is the easiest alternative therapy to master for at-home use.
An M.D., D.O., Ph.D., psychologist, or nurse with training in imagery and visualization from a state-accredited training program is the recommended provider.	Imagery and visualization are most commonly used for headaches, cancer, pain, and asthma.	Western medicine is slowly changing its view of these methods. Over a two-year period, researchers have done 30 studies involving imagery and visualization.	In the 1960s, an oncologist realized that patients with spontaneous remission of cancer were usually the ones who had always imagined themselves as being well.

(*continued*)

Approach	What It Is	How It Works	Where It Came From
Massage Therapy	Massage uses various techniques to manipulate body tissue for thera- peutic purposes.	Massage seems to work by increasing circulation and thereby relieving tension and pain, allowing toxins in the body to dissipate.	Just about every culture has practiced some form of body manipulation to ease pain and prevent or cure illness.
Meditation and Relaxation	You make a concentrated effort to focus on a phys- ical experience, sound, or thought to bring peace of mind and aid in healing.	Meditation and relaxation reduces your body's re- sponse to stress. In turn, this can improve symptoms of stress-related conditions.	Most of the techniques used today originated in ancient Eastern and Western spiritual traditions.
Music Therapy	Music is used to accom- plish therapeutic goals.	Music may stall, or even reverse, stress-related conditions and improve concentration and memory.	Throughout history, music was thought to cure plagues, alleviate mental disorders, and reduce depression.
Naturopathy	A holistic and preventive approach, it incorporates natural remedies, in- cluding Ayurvedic medi- cine, herbs, homeopathy, hydrotherapy, massage, meditation, and Tradi- tional Chinese Medicine.	N.D.'s mix and match different treatments, customizing therapy for each person and his particular health condition.	This therapy began more than a century ago when some conventional medi- cine treatments seemed extreme.
Traditional Chinese Medicine	This modality is a holistic form of medicine that utilizes herbs, diet, acupuncture, and other methods to treat and prevent health problems.	Patients are questioned and evaluated by the practitioner. A treatment or prevention program that utilizes herbs, acupuncture, diet, or exercise may be recom- mended.	Traditional Chinese Medi- cine dates back to about 476 B.C.
Yoga	This therapy is a holistic system of postures and breathing exercises meant to reunite mind, body, and breath.	The calm and well-being that yoga creates has been shown to counter the body's reaction to stress.	Yoga started as a spiri- tual discipline in India 6,000 years ago.

*A.H.G., American Herbalists Guild; B.A.M.S., Bachelor of Ayurvedic Medicine and Surgery; B.C.I.A.-C., certifica- tion from the Biofeedback Institute of America; C.C.H., Certified in Classical Homeopathy; C.M.T., certified music therapist; C.N.M.T., certified neuromuscular massage therapist; D.H.A.N.P., diplomate of the Homeopathic Academy of Naturopathic Physicians; D.Ht., diplomate in homeotherapeutics; L.Ac., licensed acupuncturist; L.M.T., licensed massage therapist; N.D., naturopathic doctor; O.M.D., doctor of Oriental medicine; O.T.R., registered occupational therapist; R.M.T., registered music therapist

Who Does It*	What It's Good For	Acceptance	Factoid
Look for an L.M.T. or a C.N.M.T.	Muscle tension, pain, and injury, and stress can all be treated with massage.	Scientific research has begun to unravel how the more than 100 massage methods work.	In different languages, massage has been referred to as *toogi-toogi*, *anmo*, and *nuad bo-rarn*.
Psychologists with a Ph.D. and O.T.R.'s are recommended.	Irritable bowel syndrome, ulcers, high blood pressure, and insomnia, and other stress-related conditions may be eased.	Doctors are prescribing meditation as a way to lower blood pressure, ease asthma, and generally relax.	Buddhists believe that meditation is essential for cultivation of wisdom and for understanding reality.
A therapist has an R.M.T. designation through the National Association for Music Therapy or a C.M.T. designation through the American Association for Music Therapy.	It alleviates stress, insomnia, and depression.	There are approximately 6,000 practitioners in the United States.	Researchers found that students who listened to a Mozart piano sonata scored higher on a test of spatial intelligence than those who sat in silence or listened to instruction.
See an expert with an N.D. degree from an accredited naturopathic medical school.	The emphasis is on health restoration, prevention, and boosting the body's natural healing process.	Studies analyzing naturopathic therapies have shown favorable results.	In 1994, Bastyr University (an accredited school of naturopathic medicine) beat out Harvard University for a hefty federal grant to study AIDS treatment.
Look for certification by the National Commission for the Certification of Acupuncture and Oriental Medicine in Washington, D.C. Experts may be L.Ac.'s or trained physicians (M.D. or D.O.) as well as O.M.D.'s.	It is effective in treating skin conditions as well as digestive problems.	The benefits of acupuncture, a component of Traditional Chinese Medicine, have been affirmed by the National Institutes of Health.	In ancient China, wealthy households retained their own herbalists, who were paid only when the households were healthy.
No national standards exist for yoga instruction. Ask the potential teacher where and for how long he has trained.	It's great for stress relief and increasing flexibility.	Although yoga seems to have a positive effect on stress, scientific study on other health problems remains mixed.	Yoga means "union" or "joining" in Sanskrit, as in joining the mind, body, and breath.

Healing Yourself

How to Get What You Need

How do you find a decent herbalist? How do you know that the acupuncturist about to stab you with multiple needles really knows what he's doing?

In conventional medicine, there's no guarantee that you won't run into an incompetent doctor, but at least you can count on every M.D. having a medical school degree and a state license. Not so in alternative medicine. The amount of official oversight to which individual therapies are subjected varies enormously. Acupuncturists are licensed in 32 states, for example; naturopaths are licensed in 14, and homeopaths in 5.

Educational standards are equally varied. In China, acupuncturists train for years. But here in the United States, there are certification programs that will give you a diploma with 50 hours of hands-on experience. Even the experts confess that the situation is not always what you'd call consumer-friendly. "It's getting better, but it's still tough out there," says Dr. Bruce Pomeranz of the University of Toronto Medical School. "I have trouble, when I'm sick, knowing which alternative guy to go to."

The Rules of Navigation

There are definitely steps you can take that will help you find an acupuncturist who knows which end of the needle is up, or a homeopath who knows that the law of similars isn't a guideline for getting lucky in a singles bar. We asked for some guidance from several people who know the alternative health care marketplace as well as anyone does, and here are their suggestions.

Ask your doctor. There's no getting around the fact that the most consistently reliable training and licensing process going at the moment is still conventional medicine's. For that reason, the most consistently reliable way of finding a qualified alternative practitioner in your area is to find a family doctor who is receptive to, and familiar with, alternative medicine. "Patients should expect that their doctors become informed enough to help guide them, and they have a right to demand that physicians do so," says Dr. James S. Gordon of the Mind/Body Center.

One way to find an M.D. in your area who is receptive to alternative medicine is to contact the American Holistic Medical Association (AHMA). Many of its members, like Kathleen Fry, M.D., a homeopathic practitioner in private practice in Scottsdale, Arizona, practice both conventional and alternative medicine or share practices with various types of alternative practitioners. You can access the AHMA's online referral directory by clicking on your browser's search button and typing "American Holistic Medical Association." Or write to the AHMA at 6728 Old McLean Village Drive, McLean, VA 22101-3906.

Another good source of information is the American Holistic Nurses Association (AHNA), which has a significantly larger membership than the AHMA (4,000 members versus 500). Holistic nurses make a point of being tied in with the alternative communities in their areas and so can be an invaluable source of information. Contact the AHNA at P. O. Box 2130, Flagstaff, AZ 86003-2130.

Call the authorities. To find out which types of therapists are licensed in your state, call the state board of medical examiners, your local or state health departments, or your local representative in the state legislature, Dr. Fry suggests.

Get online. Another invaluable source of information is the Internet. Some of the major national organizations have their own Web sites, where you'll usually find plenty of material explaining what the therapy consists of and, often, referral information. Because Web addresses change so often, we can't list them here, but a browser search using the organization's name should get you there quickly enough.

Ask a friend. Word of mouth is a surprisingly reliable way to find an alternative practitioner that you'll like, according to Dr. Gordon. "The best referrals I get in my practice come from other patients," he says. "They know who's going to work well with me because they know the kinds of things I ask patients to do and whether their friends will be ready to do it."

Grill 'em. Remember that when you agree to be treated by any health care professional, you're hiring him. And like any prospective employer, you have a right to conduct a job interview. Asking some preliminary questions over the phone can rule out the obvious rejects, but when you're getting closer to making a decision, there's really no substitute for a face-to-face visit. Doctors call that a consultation, and it's reasonable to expect to pay for it. Rates will vary, but a fee of up to $100 for an alternative practitioner would be typical, estimates Wendy Wetzel, R.N., a family nurse practitioner, certified holistic nurse, and longtime officer with the American Holistic Nurses Association. "It's well worth the expense of a consultation to see if it's somebody you can work with," she says. "If a practitioner doesn't want to do a consultation, look elsewhere."

Listen to your gut. Gathering information is important, but there's a limit to how far the just-the-facts-ma'am approach can take you. In the end, you have to rely on your instincts.

Be Prepared

When you interview an alternative practitioner, Dr. James S. Gordon of the Center for Mind/Body Medicine suggests that you ask the following questions.

- Where were you trained?
- What degrees or certificates have you earned?
- How long have you been practicing?
- What professional associations are you a member of?
- What is your healing philosophy?
- Have you been able to help people with my condition in the past? May I contact some of them?
- Is there any research that shows that this treatment works for my condition?
- How long will it take before I see results?
- Are there any potential side effects or interaction with medicine that I'm already taking or treatment that I'm already getting?
- How much will each session—and any medication/supplements/herbs—cost?

"You really have to use your intelligence and your intuition in deciding whether you want to go with any practitioner, alternative or conventional," says Dr. Gordon. "When you're asking your questions, listen to the content of the answers, but try to get a sense of what kind of person this is as well."

Keep your doc in the loop. If you're under a doctor's care for any medical condition, it's important that the lines of communication be open between your M.D. and any alternative therapist you go to. That's especially true if you're on medication and you're thinking of embarking on any course of herbal or nutritional therapy, says Dr. Fry, because a few prescription drugs can interact dangerously with such treatments. Patients undergoing chemotherapy or radiation therapy, in particular, should exercise caution.

Growing Your Own

Herb Gardening Made Easy

A lot of nuts-and-berries types will tell you that it all went sour for America about the time we replaced horseflesh with horsepower. Once upon a time, we communed with the land, the lecture goes. Now we commune only with our laptops.

We'll spare you the guilt trip. And we won't tell you that you're an awful person simply because your deepest connection with the soil comes from sliding into second base during softball season. We *are* going to tell you that you might be missing out on something fun and healthy—and perhaps more satisfying than you ever thought possible.

A Harvest of Healing

You already know that herbal remedies are among the broadest, deepest, most important reservoirs available to practitioners of alternative healing. But the healing isn't just in the harvesting; it's in the growing, the cultivating. And that's the easy part. "Anybody who plants a basic herb garden is going to feel like a genuine gardener pretty quickly," says Scott Meyer, a senior editor for *Organic Gardening* magazine and an avid gardener for more than 10 years. "The truth is that a lot of herbs are like weeds. If you rip them out of your garden and throw them down on the ground and stomp on them, they'll grow again. You couldn't get rid of them if you wanted to."

Not that you'll want to. As you'll find, there's something undeniably fulfilling about growing, harvesting, and consuming an herb you've raised yourself, especially when that herb makes you feel better. So, with fun and good health in mind, here's a down-in-the-dirt guide to starting a simple backyard garden with four of the most useful (and easy-to-grow) medicinal herbs.

Garlic. You might not realize it, but that immune-bolstering garlic bulb in your kitchen is a seed. Buy a planting bulb or two from a nursery (the supermarket variety may not be as hardy) in October or November. Dig a furrow about 6 to 8 inches deep and eight feet long. Take a bulb apart and plant individual cloves, pointy side up, about 10 inches to a foot apart. Don't peel the skin off the cloves; it protects them from mold. Fill in the furrow loosely with moist dirt and cover it with mulch, straw, or dry grass clippings to keep away weeds.

If it's a dry winter, keep the ground around your garlic plantings a bit moist. In the spring, shoots will come up. Harvest a few if you like—they have a mild garlic flavor—but not all. You'll know the garlic is ready when the leaves start to turn yellow, in June or July, depending on the climate. For each clove you planted, you should now have a full-size bulb. Dig them up carefully (you don't want to damage the bulbs with your shovel) and cure them by hanging them in a cool, dry place for about a month.

Peppermint. This stomach-problem soother grows in the early spring, anytime the temperature is past 65°F. You need to grow mint plants from other mint plants, not from seeds. Get a cutting from a friend or a started plant from a gardening store. A cutting is a leaf with its stem still attached. Put the stem in a glass of water for about a week until roots start to grow. If you decide to use a cutting, start it growing indoors, on a sunny

TAKE 2 EACH DAY

windowsill. Get some potting soil from a hardware store or nursery (potting soil is specially mixed to give new plants a strong head start) and loosely fill a small pot about the size of an empty yogurt container (roughly four inches across at the lip). Stick the stem of your peppermint plant in and cover it with soil up to where the first leaf begins. Keep it moist, and in about three weeks, you'll see new leaves sprouting from the stem. When it has three full-size leaves, it's time to take it outside.

Dig a hole just slightly larger than the container your peppermint plant is in. Remove the dirt and loosen it up with your fingers. Put your peppermint seedling in the hole, cover it up with soil to the lowest leaf, water it occasionally if you're not getting rain, and within a month you'll have an established plant. That's when you can start using the leaves, but don't take more than a third of the leaves at any one time. Peppermint, which will return each year in most North American climates, can be invasive and should be kept under control by regularly cutting it back.

Rosemary. Unlike peppermint, you can grow this memory-improving herb from seeds. Get them at a nursery. To plant, moisten the ground a bit—the soil should be loose enough to stick your finger in without too much difficulty. Dig a hole that's about as deep as the second knuckle on your pinkie finger. Drop two seeds in, move six inches on, and do it again. Fill the holes in loosely with soil until they're parallel with the ground—don't mound the soil up or pack it in. You should see sprouts in about two weeks. Or, if you're the impatient type, forgo the seeds (they take a long time to grow) and buy a started plant at a nursery.

Rosemary plants are more vulnerable to weed encroachment than peppermint is, especially in their younger days, so make sure that you keep the ground around them tidy. It's not a bad idea to surround all your plants with a

---

Self-Preservation

According to retired botanist Dr. James A. Duke in *The Green Pharmacy*, if you intend to preserve your herbs for future use, you need to dry them. Here's how.

- **Collect each herb in its own brown paper bag (not plastic). Write the name of the herb and the date you picked it on the outside.**
- **Check them in a week. If they're not drying in the bag, spread them out on newspapers or a screen in a dry, shaded area.**
- **Once they're dry—papery and crumbly—you can store them in jars or plastic bags. Keep them in a cool, dark place like a cellar or cupboard. Avoid exposing them to heat.**

---

little ground cover—grass clippings work well, or buy some mulch—to help keep weeds from threatening young stems. (Ground cover shuts off sunlight, which even weeds need to grow.) Rosemary doesn't like the soil too wet, so make doubly sure that it gets good drainage. Daily sprinklings of water are good for the seedlings. Go to deeper waterings (an inch or so a week) as the plants grow above a foot. Rosemary must usually be replanted each year.

St.-John's-wort. Buy a plant of this increasingly popular antidepressant at the nursery or get a cutting from a friend and follow the same planting procedure you did with the peppermint. This is an especially aggressive weed that also returns each year, so keep it a foot away from your other plants and be ready to cut it back when it starts to creep. In fact, St.-John's-wort is so aggressive that it's against the law to grow it in some states. Check with your nursery to make sure of its legal status where you live.

St.-John's-wort flowers in late June through August, and it's the flowers you're after, not the leaves. Wait until they open, then snip them all off. That will encourage the plant to produce another batch.

In the Store

A Consumer's Guide to Natural Remedies

It's a jungle in there. Anyone who has ever taken a walk through the herbal remedies aisles of their local health food store or drugstore knows that. A seemingly endless variety of concoctions clutters the shelves, each shouting a litany of inexplicable claims and promises: "Dried juice from young barley leaves." "Ecologically wildcrafted." "Twenty green foods supercharged with global algae." "Cryogenically ground immediately prior to cold-process percolation."

If you're overwhelmed, mystified, and suspicious, you're in good company.

"I have 60 years of herbal experience, and I have trouble figuring it out," says retired botanist Dr. James A. Duke. "It's bewildering."

Determined to find some way to sort through the chaos, we asked two of the world's top herb experts, Dr. Duke and Varro E. Tyler, Ph.D., distinguished professor emeritus of pharmacognosy and dean emeritus of Purdue University School of Pharmacy and Pharmacal Sciences in West Lafayette, Indiana, for their advice in choosing where and how to buy herbal remedies. Here are their recommendations.

Do your homework. The basic rule of alternative medicine applies to buying over-the-counter natural remedies: You have to take your own health care in hand. In this case, that means educating yourself on herbs, learning not only which herbs are best for a given purpose but also how much of a particular herb to use

and in what form. "I would read everything possible about an herb before I used it," says Dr. Tyler.

A good place to start is in the chapter The Power of Herbs on page 64 of this book. If you want more information, check out *The Green Pharmacy* by Dr. Duke, *Herbal Medicine*, by Rudolph F. Weiss; and Dr. Tyler's *Herbs of Choice* or *The Honest Herbal* at your local library or bookstore, Dr. Duke recommends.

In addition to books, most consumer health publications have regular articles on herbs these days, and the Internet is replete with herb-related Web sites. Some sources of information in both media, of course, are more reliable than others. The same goes for books and pamphlets, especially those produced by commercial interests. Be especially careful when dealing with information from the Internet. "There's a whole lot of literature out there that's intended to sell product rather than to inform accurately," says Dr. Tyler. "You want to avoid the former and seek out the latter."

Find a resource. The second phase of your herbal self-education should be finding a live person who can help answer your specific questions. "Connect with a buddy if you can," says Dr. Duke. "Establish a pipeline." That could be a knowledgeable friend, or, if you're looking to treat a specific medical condition, it could mean finding a good homeopath or naturopath.

Hit the health food store. Although you can find natural remedies in drugstores and grocery stores these days, Dr. Tyler and Dr. Duke recommend shopping for herbs in a health food store first. You'll stand a greater chance of finding a salesperson who knows and cares about the remedies on the shelf. Of course, there's no guarantee that the salesperson will know arnica from arsenic, so be sure to use a smidgen of your own common sense when getting advice from store help.

Be a pest. When you get to the store, don't be afraid to ask lots of questions. "Ask the clerk what he would take for something," says Dr. Duke. "And once he tells you, ask him why, immediately, before he has time to think about it." Flippant answers are a bad sign, Dr. Duke says. Look for retailers who are thoughtful in addition to being well-informed. If necessary, ask the clerk to call the manufacturer, or call the manufacturer yourself. "Ask why his product is better than somebody else's," Dr. Duke says. "If he doesn't have a ready answer, it may not be."

Take a standardized test. One of the most confusing aspects of buying herbs is deciding which of the many forms they come in is the best for your particular needs. Should you buy fresh herbs and make tea, or take capsules, or buy tinctures and extracts? There aren't simple answers to those questions. Some herbs work better as teas; some don't work at all as teas. Some herbs lose their potency if they are dried; others lose their potency if they are processed into tinctures. Sorting through the maze requires both knowledge and advice.

One shortcut advocated by both Dr. Tyler and Dr. Duke is to buy herbs in "standardized" dosages. What that means is that the manufacturer has processed the herb mixture contained in the capsule, to ensure that it contains a specified amount of the herb's active medicinal ingredient.

Go with quality. There are definitely right ways and wrong ways to process herbs for sale, and poorly handled herbs can be nearly worthless. Therefore, it's worth buying herbal

Buyer Beware

Don't want to waste your money on natural remedies that don't work? Here are four that Dr. Varro E. Tyler of Purdue University School of Pharmacy and Pharmacal Sciences says don't do what they're often advertised as doing: alfalfa, for arthritis; burdock, as a blood purifier; damiana, as an aphrodisiac; and suma, as a tonic. If you see them at your local store, think twice before buying them.

Dr. Tyler also lists five herbs that he believes are downright dangerous: coltsfoot, suggested as a cough suppressant (Dr. Tyler believes that it's carcinogenic); comfrey, often suggested for wound healing (another carcinogen, according to Dr. Tyler); germander, for weight loss (Dr. Tyler says that it causes liver damage); sassafras, a tonic (yet another carcinogen, says Dr. Tyler); and yohimbine, an aphrodisiac (it increases blood pressure and causes rapid heartbeat; can sometimes cause nausea and vomiting). He says that they should not be used without the guidance of an herbal expert.

products from reliable, experienced companies. Here, too, health food stores—particularly those that have been in business for a long time—are more likely to know and rely on reputable suppliers than are stores that don't consider herbs a core business. Among herbal companies trusted by Dr. Duke are Solaray, Nature's Way, Nature's Herbs, and Eclectic Institute.

Avoid the bargain basement. Because of the careful handling that herbs require to preserve their medicinal properties, a good herbal product is often going to be more expensive than one that has been cranked out of an herb mill, says Dr. Duke. In other words, in most cases, you'll get what you pay for.

Don't play doctor. Because herbal remedies are more readily available than prescription drugs, there's a temptation to take them without benefit of medical advice. Dr. Duke recommends against this. Herbs can have side effects, they can create allergic reactions, and they can interact badly with each other or with prescription drugs. Check with your physician before embarking on any course of herbal treatment: Medical diagnosis is not a sport for amateurs.

Don't believe everything you read. There is a barrage of questionable, sometimes dangerous hype out there. Dr. Duke recommends carefully reading the labels to glean as much information as possible, keeping an eye on any fillers, chemicals, or other agents used in processing. People with alcoholism may want to avoid alcohol-based tinctures, for example. Pay attention to recommended dosages, too: Sometimes the cheapest product requires two or three times the number of capsules to equal one capsule of another brand.

Go single. Many herbal products today are blends of several herbs—sometimes more than a dozen. Dr. Duke advises caution here. Although some traditional herb combinations have been used successfully for thousands of years, newer mixes have not been proved. And in both cases, research is not as widely available as it is for many single herbs. "The more herbal ingredients there are in a complex formula, the less the likelihood of any good scientific studies," Dr. Duke says.

Get fresh. Freshness counts in herbal products. Even tinctures and dried herbs lose potency over time. Dr. Tyler suggests shopping in a store that has a lot of customers, if possible. Consistent turnover means that you won't be buying an herb that has been gathering dust on the shelf for a year. Some products have expiration dates, but Dr. Tyler doesn't put much stock in them. Too much guesswork goes into assigning those dates, he says.

Be patient. Don't expect herbs to work as quickly as prescription drugs, or as dramatically, says Dr. Tyler. The healing process of herbs is more subtle and usually takes longer.

What's Your Pleasure?

We wouldn't go so far as to call herbs multimedia remedies, but the fact is that you can get them to work for you in a lot of different ways. Here are the most common methods for utilizing herbal products.

Teas. Teas are made from fresh or dried herbs. The latter are more potent because they contain less water, making the active ingredients more concentrated. Herb teas can be either infusions or decoctions. Infusions are made by pouring hot water over a tea bag or loose herbs and steeping for 5 to 10 minutes. Decoctions are made by simmering the herbs in water for 15 to 30 minutes. Decoctions are best for roots or stems, which yield their healing chemicals more reluctantly than do leaves and flowers.

Capsules. Capsules contain herb material that has been crushed into powder and placed in capsules.

Tinctures. Tinctures, also known as extracts, are made by soaking fresh herbs for days or weeks in alcohol with varying amounts of water. The mixture is then shaken, strained, and bottled for use. Tinctures are usually taken mixed in a little water.

Creams. Herbal creams and ointments are available for external use from health food stores and should be applied according to the label instructions.

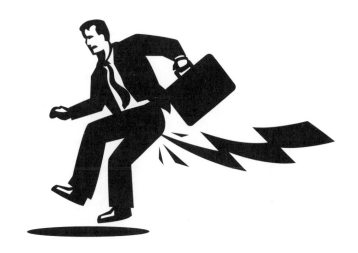

Part Two

Unleashing Your
Healing Power

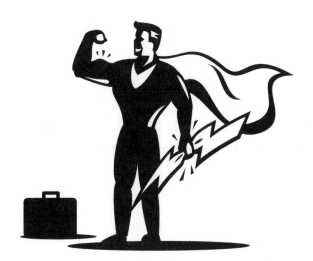

The Path to Power

Psych Yourself Up

Okay, we've given you the lay of the land. Now, it's time to take the plunge.

This section is devoted to showing you how to start putting into practice—into your life—the various alternative healing arts we've talked about so far. We have lots of practical suggestions, all designed to help you harness the power of holistic health care. Some of them will seem a little odd; others may seem downright ridiculous. To paraphrase a well-known explorer of exotic territories, you may suspect you're not in Kansas anymore.

As preparation for the journey, there are four key qualities of character we suggest that you include in your psychic supply kit.

An open mind. This is the probably the single most important quality to have as you head out on the alternative highway. It's especially important to keep in mind when confronting things that seem inexplicable.

Many alternative therapies, especially those imported from the East, arrive embedded in unfamiliar philosophies. You do not—repeat, do not—have to buy into the belief systems underlying any of these therapies in order to benefit from the alternative health practices they've produced.

"Studies have been done in which subjects were asked how much they believed in the treatments they received," says Bruce Pomeranz, M.D., Ph.D., a neurophysiologist at the University of Toronto Medical

School and a leading researcher into the physiological effects of acupuncture. "There was very low correlation between belief and outcome. I think if you're hostile to these methods, you will turn them off, so you should at least try to be open. But you don't have to be a true believer."

Having an open mind can also save you a lot of needless suffering. Many believers in alternative medicine became believers only because they developed serious health problems that conventional medicine couldn't fix. They turned to acupuncture or meditation or homeopathy as a last resort. "The vast majority of patients I see have been to anywhere from 4 to 10 conventional doctors," says M. Kyu Chung, M.D., a certified acupuncturist and chief of family medicine at Cooper Health Systems in Camden, New Jersey.

That's a shame, because one of the strongest selling points of alternative medicine is that it can keep people from getting sick in the first place. Give those preventive powers a shot *before* your body's ailing.

An adventurous spirit. There are guys who think nothing of skydiving or shark hunting but who likely would be terrified—okay, dubious, at least—of going to an aromatherapist or a naturopath. As a result, many holistic health practitioners will tell you that they see far more women than they do men. "Our practice is 75 percent women," says David Edelberg, M.D., chairman and founder of American WholeHealth, a holistic health center in Chicago. "Typically, the wife comes in and has a positive experience. A few weeks later, she drags in the old man, kicking and screaming."

Men's notorious reluctance to visit any doctor only partly explains that gender skew, in Dr. Edelberg's opinion. Alternative medicine is especially challenging for many men, he says, because so much of it is based on the conviction that people's emotions have a profound influence on their health. Dealing with feelings is not a masculine strong suit, Dr. Edelberg believes. "Men tend to regard their bodies the same way that they regard their carburetors," he says. "If something is wrong, they want somebody to go in there, fix it, and close it back up. Purely mechanics."

Getting the benefits of alternative medicine requires more active, and often more thoughtful, participation. It requires, in short, a sense of adventure. You have that, haven't you?

A gambler's heart. We've acknowledged it before and we'll acknowledge it again: Not all of the therapies in this book are backed up by the kind of scientific studies that conventional medicine likes to claim as proof that a particular treatment is 100 percent reliable. But don't let that lack of definitive research stop you.

We're not suggesting that you abandon all of your critical faculties. What we're saying is that the American health care system is going through a transition period of historic proportions. Conventional medicine is only beginning to take seriously some of these alternative approaches to healing. In many alternative fields, new research is under way. Some forms of therapy, such as acupuncture, have already been scientifically vindicated. Others, such as prayer, are extremely difficult to quantify, even when much of the available research suggests that they do work.

The point is that conventional scientific research is not necessarily the only acceptable evidence. Empirical evidence—the evidence of personal experience—is also an acceptable standard. If an alternative therapy works for you, it has value, regardless of what the scientists say.

That's true, in part, because many of these therapies are benign, meaning that they won't cause damage in and of themselves. Postponing proper medical treatment when such treatment can arrest or cure a serious health condition *can* cause damage, however. If you suspect that you have such a condition, definitely get it checked out by the best medical doctor you can find. But if you're healthy, or if you think an alternative treatment may work for a condition that isn't critical, give it a try, says Dr. Edelberg. In many cases, that's the only way we learn.

An investigator's instinct. It's possible to be adventurous and still keep your eyes open. With the ever-increasing interest in alternative remedies, inevitably there are going to be people with an interest in separating you from your hard-earned cash in return for remedies or treatment that they're either not fully qualified to give or that simply don't work.

So as you enter this environment, think of yourself as an investigator. Make Sherlock Holmes your model. Be skeptical, be smart, and be ready to challenge traditional assumptions and assertions.

Earlier in the book, we offered a primer on how to find a legitimate alternative practitioner. One point bears repeating, though. Being a pioneer requires more than the usual amount of diligence and preparation. "Be your own advocate," says Sheila Quinn, executive director of the American Association of Naturopathic Physicians in Seattle. "If you were looking for care for a relative or friend, you would ask lots of questions and get lots of information before you made a recommendation. Do as much for yourself."

That means making a few visits to the local health food store before you actually buy anything. That means quizzing alternative practitioners before you ever agree to whatever treatment they practice. That means perusing the literature—including this book and others—to answer the questions that will naturally pop up as you explore alternatives. The goal is for you to be comfortable and accepting—the more you are, the more these techniques and practices will work. And they do work.

Go along now and start exploring. The path beckons before you.

The Power of the Mind

If You Think You're Healthy, You're Right

Modern life is fraught with tensions, insecurities, conflicts, and frustrations. That's inevitable. It's how we handle those tensions, insecurities, conflicts, and frustrations that makes the difference and that keeps us healthy. Those who study the human mind believe that many of us have a natural propensity for negativity. Our emotions, they say, can easily get stuck in patterns of anger, resentment, discouragement, and cynicism. And these negative emotions can deal a major blow to your health. They raise your stress levels, which can raise blood pressure and put you at greater risk for problems like heart disease. They depress your immune system, leaving you more susceptible to a raft of illnesses, from the common cold to cancer.

As it happens, some believe that the reverse is just as true. Learn to turn those negative emotions around, learn to laugh at stress, learn to take charge of your own thoughts and feelings, and you can literally think yourself well.

Stinking Thinking

In the 1960s, a psychologist named Aaron T. Beck, M.D., began to investigate a curious phenomenon that he had noticed: Depressed people seemed to see themselves as losers even though their actual achievements often suggested that they were anything but.

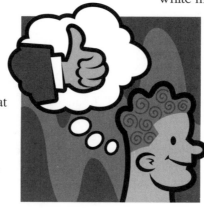

As Dr. Beck explored further, he discovered that many people, for a variety of reasons, develop "a systematic bias" in perception that causes them to expect the worst—an expectation that all too often becomes a self-fulfilling prophecy. Over the years, he and his colleagues developed a list of the more common types of "thinking errors" into which many of us fall. You might call them negativity's "greatest hits."

- Catastrophizing: A propensity for believing the worst-case scenario. For example, "If the boss doesn't like my report, I will be instantly fired."
- All-or-nothing thinking: The tendency to see things in black-and-white dichotomies. "If I don't win this tennis match, I'll be a failure."
- Discounting the positive: "Something good happened? A fluke."
- Emotional reasoning: The belief that just because you feel something, it must be so.
- Labeling: Whatever moves, slap a label on it, usually a negative label. "He got promoted? He must be a brownnoser."
- Mental filtering: To paraphrase singer-songwriter Paul Simon, men hear only what they want to hear; they disregard everything else.
- Mind reading: You know what she's thinking, and you don't like it.
- Overgeneralization: All bosses are scum. White men can't jump.
- Should and must statements: "You must do it my way or else."
- Personalization: "That pretty girl crossed the street just now to avoid me."

All of us have, to greater or lesser degrees, a tendency for leaping to these kinds of mental conclusions, says Michelle G. Newman, Ph.D., assistant professor of psychology at Pennsylvania State University in University Park. The problems come when they become ingrained, entrenched thought patterns. "Every time you make a negative prediction, your body reacts as though that prediction really happened," she says. "So you feel sad or anxious, as if it really did happen. You're essentially creating chronic unhappiness."

Eliminating the Negative

To defeat the thinking patterns that create chronic unhappiness, it helps to have a set of mental tools that can stop negative thoughts in their tracks. You can train your mind to use those tools, much as you would train your body to perform athletically. "You don't wait until it's the end of the basketball game and your team is behind by one point to start practicing your free throws," says Redford B. Williams, M.D., director of Behavioral Medicine Research at Duke University Medical Center in Durham, North Carolina, and co-author of two books on emotion and health, *Anger Kills* and *Lifeskills.* "You practice and practice and practice, day in and day out, when nobody is around, so that when the game is on the line, you can increase your chances of making that crucial basket."

With that advice in mind, we've assembled a list of drills that will help you master the fundamentals of emotional well-being.

Know your triggers. All of us have emotional triggers that can set off our negative thinking patterns. Learning what they are will help us keep our emotional safety switches on. "It pays to become a detective of your

Be a Visionary

Creating and nurturing a restful or reassuring mental vision can impart a peaceful state of mind, which, in turn, can communicate a sense of relaxation throughout the body. Two legal ways of doing this are called visualization and imagery.

Visualization is the simpler of the two, according to Dennis C. Turk, Ph.D., John and Emma Bonica professor of anesthesiology and pain research at the University of Washington School of Medicine in Seattle. The idea is to picture a scene in your mind. It could be a mental movie of yourself acing an upcoming job interview, or a highlight film of yourself sinking a tricky putt on the 15th green.

Imagery involves imagining a more fully developed, multimedia scenario, replete not only with sights but also with smells, tastes, sounds, and textures. The idea is not so much to picture yourself completing a task but to put yourself in another place for awhile. Dr. Turk often encourages his patients to imagine themselves walking through a meadow on a warm summer day, feeling the grass beneath their feet and a light breeze on their skin, hearing birds chirping nearby. Then he suggests that they imagine themselves lying down beneath a tree, half in the sun and half in the shade, feeling the sun and the grass and perhaps tasting some sweet-tangy lemonade. The multiplicity of sensory elements involved in such a scene, Dr. Turk says, tends to be deeply engaging, which is why imagery works so well.

What does it work for? Besides helping people relax, imagery can help distract from pain, while visualization can be an effective way to rehearse success rather than failure, Dr. Turk says.

own behavior," says Carla Perez, M.D., a psychiatrist in private practice in San Francisco who has written extensively on controlling compulsive behavior. "You have to know who the enemy is before you can go after it. Pay attention to what sets you off."

Take notes. Keeping a record of your emotional ups and downs—by writing them down in a journal, say—is an excellent tool for learning what makes you tick emotionally, Dr. Perez suggests. On a daily basis, carefully track what feelings and experiences set off different kinds of reactions. Describe them specifically. Over time, your patterns will become obvious.

Assess the situation. When confronted with a situation that pushes your emotional buttons, Dr. Williams recommends asking yourself the following questions: Is it important? Is the reaction I'm having appropriate to the facts of the actual situation? Is there anything I can do about it?

If the answer to all three is yes, then ask yourself one last question: Is it worth it to take whatever action would be necessary to change the situation?

Many times the answer to that last question will be no, Dr. Williams says. For example, your boss may be acting inappropriately in ways that have a significant impact on your work life and on your emotions, but telling him to take a flying leap probably isn't going to serve your best interests in the long run. You may, however, want to start looking for another job. "If the answer to all four questions is yes, then you must take some action," says Dr. Williams. The trick is making sure that action is an appropriate one.

Count to 10. Finding some way to distract yourself, whether it be reciting the Ten Commandments or thinking about your favorite Rolling Stones song, is one of the oldest, best methods of dealing with disturbing emotions—anger, in particular. Dr. Williams calls distraction a way of "short-circuiting the hostility cascade."

Find support. Twelve-step programs have helped millions of people deal with a host of different addictions and compulsive patterns,

and numerous research studies have shown that being part of a supportive social environment enhances health. The message is clear, says Dr. Perez: Talking about your problems with people who truly understand from their own firsthand experiences is good for you. Look around until you find a group you feel comfortable in, but don't let the awkwardness of being a newcomer scare you off prematurely, she suggests.

Meditate. You don't have to be "spiritual" to get plenty of help from sitting in a quiet place for a few minutes every day and concentrating on the rhythm of your breathing. The key is learning how to temporarily quiet the mind's incessant chatter in order to gain a respite from the stresses of everyday life, writes Herbert Benson, M.D., associate professor of medicine at Harvard Medical School and president of the Mind/Body Medical Institute at New England Deaconess Hospital in Boston, in his book *Timeless Healing*. A belief in God is not a prerequisite, according to Dr. Benson.

Getting Feedback

There has always been something creepy about being hooked up with sensors to a machine: images of *1984* and *A Clockwork Orange* come to mind. But in the science known as biofeedback, the machines you'd be hooked up to would be there not to control you in some totalitarian nightmare but to enable you to become more in control of yourself. "It's a way to teach you about your body," says Dr. Dennis C. Turk of the University of Washington School of Medicine. "After doing biofeedback, you'll realize that you have a lot more control over your body than you may have thought. You can learn how to mentally make changes in body processes associated with stress and pain."

There are three basic types of biofeedback, all of which measure stress. One, the most common, measures muscle tension; another measures brain waves; a third measures temperature. (The temperature in your fingertips rises or lowers depending on how stressed you are.) In each case, sensors are attached to your body—in different places, depending on what kind of tension is being monitored—which convey information in the form of electrical impulses to a little machine. This information is displayed in either audio or visual form. If it's an audio biofeedback machine, you will hear a series of clicks or beeps, which will increase in speed depending on how tense you are. A visual machine will display the readings on a monitor as a line graph or as a light that gets brighter or dimmer. In either case, the point is to give you an objective reading of exactly what your body is doing at that moment. It's a lot like a Geiger counter, only a biofeedback machine measures tension instead of radiation.

After getting used to the way the machine responds to your body, you'll be encouraged to experiment with various types of relaxation techniques—deep breathing, meditation, visualization, prayer, whatever—to see what works best for you. The machine provides very specific feedback on how your body is responding, which is why it's called a biofeedback machine.

The vast majority of people who try biofeedback learn what they need to learn in six sessions, Dr. Turk says. Be suspicious of anyone who tries to sell you on a longer series of treatments. Each session usually consists of about a half-hour on the machine. To find a certified biofeedback therapist in your area, Dr. Turk recommends asking your family doctor for a referral. Or for a free list of certified biofeedback therapists in the United States, you can contact the Association for Applied Psychophysiology and Biofeedback, 10200 West 44th Avenue, Suite 304, Wheat Ridge, CO 80033-2840.

Affirm Yourself

Thanks in large part to Stuart Smalley, affirmations have acquired a pretty wimpy reputation. Smalley was the lisping loser (played for several seasons on *Saturday Night Live* by comedian Al Franken) who always looked into a mirror to reassure himself, "Goshdarnit, people like me."

As simpering as Smalley seemed, many therapists still believe that affirmations can be a useful countermeasure for fighting the negative messages we tend to tell ourselves. Dr. Carla Perez, a psychiatrist in San Francisco, recommends finding a peaceful spot in a park or a comfortable chair at home and telling yourself statements such as, "I feel good about myself and my life" or "Only I know what I want in my life"—whatever fits your particular issues. It's not necessary to utter such statements out loud, she says, although doing so will make them more emphatic. Writing them down helps, too.

The real audience for affirmations is the unconscious mind, where the master tapes that we want to record over are buried. "You need to demolish all the pessimistic, doubting parts of your psyche that have been given too much power in the past," says Dr. Perez.

Besides teaching people how to relax, biofeedback is mainly used for teaching how to control various types of pain, especially headache pain, neck pain, and back pain. Dr. Turk emphasizes, however, that sensors can tell you only about symptoms, not causes. "It's important to look at whatever factors have contributed to the symptoms in the first place," he says. For example, if your neck muscles get tense every time you talk about your partner, then in addition to reducing the tension in your neck muscles, you may also want to focus on what's going on in your relationship.

The Power of the Spirit

Plugging In to a Higher Power

A lot of serious scientists have been spending a lot of time and money in past years applying rational principles of research to see if it's possible to determine whether religion has a measurable impact on health. And they've come up with some pretty interesting results. For example:

- A large study of people in Maryland found that those who attended church once a week or more had lower death rates from heart disease, emphysema, cirrhosis of the liver, and suicide than those who did not.
- A study of heart patients at San Francisco General Medical Center found that those who were prayed for—without their knowledge— were less likely to suffer complications than those who were not prayed for.

Another body of research has documented the health benefits of meditation. Studies have found that:

- Patients with high blood pressures who meditated experienced significant drops in their blood pressures and needed fewer or no medications.
- Patients with chronic pain who meditated experienced less severity of pain, less anxiety, less depression, and less anger. They were also more active.

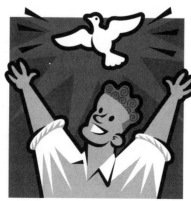

Consistent as these findings are, some mystery remains as to what, exactly, causes those benefits. Do people who pray, for example, get better because God has answered their prayers or because they believe he will? Are churchgoers healthier because they are blessed with holy grace or because their social group tends to smoke less, drink less, and take their medicines more regularly?

Researchers acknowledge that community support and healthier lifestyles are part of the answer, as is the calm, accepting attitude that characterizes meditation. Whether those social and psychological effects are the whole story is something research is unlikely to ever uncover.

"We can ponder the tantalizing idea of divine intervention, but it remains ultimately unprovable because it requires faith, which is in a different category than science," says Dale Matthews, M.D., associate professor of internal medicine at Georgetown University Medical Center in Washington, D.C., and one of the leading researchers into the health-religion connection.

Making Prayer Work for You

It's hard to say how strongly a person has to believe in order for faith to improve his health. At least one of the major researchers in the field—Dr. Herbert Benson of Harvard Medical School—asserts that you don't have to believe in God at all. That position may raise some eyebrows in religious circles, but it's safe to say that few religious leaders would question the proposition that any spiritual seeker can increase his faith by practicing prayer.

Prayer is perhaps most simply defined as having a conversation with God. Of course, definitions of the "G" word vary enormously. Whatever your definition, here are some basic strategies that Dr. Matthews suggests for putting the power of prayer to work in your life.

Develop a relationship. The key to an effective prayer life, Dr. Matthews explains, is developing a sense that you have an ongoing relationship with God. "If we conceive of God as a friend we can talk to any time, about anything," he writes in his book *The Faith Factor: Proof of the Healing Power of Prayer*, "or if we meditate on the nature of God and his goodness, we are likely to find a deep sense of satisfaction and even joy in our prayer and in our lives."

Set aside some time. Prayer is like anything else you tend to do for yourself: It can get pushed aside by other seemingly more pressing commitments. Don't let that happen. Many people like to start and end their day with prayer. Prayer books that have a scripture or thought for each day of the year have become popular in providing a focus for those times. Going on retreats for more extended periods of prayer and reflection is another popular route to maintaining a spiritual connection, says Dr. Matthews.

Make a sacred place. Find a spot where you can pray comfortably and without interruption. Creating a special "prayer corner" with a few spiritual objects or pictures can put you in a prayerful mood, says Dr. Matthews.

Pray on the run. Specific prayer times are the foundation of a healthy prayer life, but praying spontaneously—in line at the grocery store, for example, or while you're doing the dishes—is a skill worth cultivating, says Dr. Matthews.

Find a mentor. Neophyte spiritual seekers may want to apprentice themselves to more seasoned guides, says Dr. Matthews. "Go under the wing of someone who is more experienced in the faith," he says. Most religious congregations make it a point to have prayer and spiritual growth groups or even coffee hours or other social activities where potential mentors can be found.

Find a community. The health benefits of consistent participation in a supportive community, religious and otherwise, have been thoroughly documented. Not coincidentally, sharing the religious experience with others is a central element of most faith traditions. People who tend to find conventional churchgoing too impersonal can find a more intimate sense of connection by joining one of the small scripture or prayer discussion groups that are becoming increasingly popular in many congregations today, Dr. Matthews suggests.

Meditating Yourself

Meditation, or meditative prayer, is less about talking to God and more about listening, less about conversation and more about awareness. It's a conscious attempt to still the ceaseless chatter of thoughts that typically fills our heads, day in and day out. Meditators shift to a less distracted, more peaceful, and more spiritually connected state of consciousness.

Dr. Benson has observed a form of secularized meditation that he calls the relaxation response. Learning to practice the relaxation response is a surprisingly simple process that, according to Dr. Benson, consists mainly of two basic steps.

1. Find a focus. The essence of meditation is training the mind to focus, and having something to focus on—a word, a sound, a prayer, a phrase, or an activity—can help. Jogging, swimming, and even knitting qualify. Dr. Benson recommends these as secular focus words: *one, ocean, love, peace, calm,* or *relax*. As religious focus words or prayers, he suggests *Our Father, who art in heaven; Lord Jesus Christ, have mercy on me; shalom;* or *om*.

2. Disregard interruptions. When everyday thoughts try to intrude on your focus, as they inevitably will, impassively put them out of your mind and return, gently, to your focus, says Dr. Benson.

Those are the basic tools you'll need to start meditating.

The Power of Sight

What You See Is What You Get

It makes perfect sense that when God wanted to set all of creation rolling, one of the first things he did was turn on the light. Few forces in our world possess as much intrinsic, pervasive power as light, and the information it brings to our eyes has a dramatic impact on our bodies and our minds. Consider this: You see an attractive woman walk down the street; the old soldier twinges. View the sun setting over the ocean or rising above a mountain; stress melts away and you feel relaxed, contemplative. Round a curve in the road and see a major traffic jam ahead; you feel anger and despair. Watch the shower scene in *Psycho*; your pulse races and your stomach churns.

Sight clearly works both ways: It can make us feel better, physically and mentally, or it can make us feel worse. To the degree that we can emphasize the former and downplay the latter, the happier and healthier we'll be. There are two basic areas in which we can use the power of sight to affect our health, one having to do with the amount of light we need, the other having to do with the nature of the visual stimuli we take in. Here's a snapshot of each approach.

A Sight for Sore Eyes

It's not only the quantity of the light around us that has an effect but also what that light reveals. Our environment has a huge impact on our state of mind and, therefore, on our health. Sight is probably our predominant means of taking in information on that environment. It makes

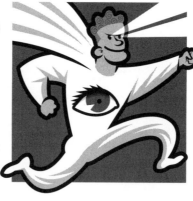

sense, then, to see that what we're consuming visually is good for us. Here's how.

Color me mellow. Research has shown that the colors of walls and other interior surfaces can have a decided impact on mood. You can put that knowledge into use in your own surroundings, says Cam Busch, R.N., a certified art therapist in Chattanooga, Tennessee. Incorporate softer colors—lighter blues, greens, mauves, and eggshell white—in places where you're stressed. Use brighter colors in rooms where you want to be more upbeat and energetic. Red and orange, for example, are known as stimulating colors.

Go natural. It's no accident that Ansel Adams is a big seller in the office art department. Pictures of nature tend to have a restorative effect on our state of mind, so find a big wall calendar with a picture of a different landscape for each month and tack it to your wall. Or hang a print of your favorite natural setting, suggests Deborah Good, Ph.D., chairwoman of the art therapy program at Southwestern College in Santa Fe, New Mexico, and president of the American Art Therapy Association, which is headquartered in Mundelein, Illinois. Dr. Good once worked in a prison where the inmates painted a wall mural of a forest scene with streams running through it. "When you entered the room, it looked like you were outside," she says, "which was very healing for the prisoners because they couldn't get outside." Hopefully, your office isn't quite that confining, but a nature scene may still help you feel a little less trapped behind your desk.

Create peaceful pictures. Use a camera to create some nature pictures of your own, suggests Busch. "Taking photographs is a way to bring the outer image and the inner meaning together," she says, "and it gives you a record of that experience that you can always refer back to."

Get out. If Mother Nature is the consummate artist, taking walks in natural settings may be the best visual remedy of all. Try to get out to a local park or nearby scenic vista at least once a week to drink it in. While walking or enjoying the view, Busch recommends listening carefully to the thoughts that emerge "from the silence" and putting them down in a journal. That can create another form of record, like a photograph, that will help to re-create the experience for you at times when you can't get out and enjoy the real thing.

Hang an artist. Kings and billionaires may not just be showing off: Having art on the walls has therapeutic value. You don't have to know a lot about art to pick a soothing print to hang on your wall; you just have to know what you like. Go to a frame shop or art store and treat yourself to a print. As you look at the selections, pay attention to how you feel when you set eyes on each of the different images, suggests Dr. Good. A scribbly Picasso or neon-hued Warhol may only remind you how busy and fast-paced your life is. A plump Botticelli nude or florid Monet landscape may soothe you—or simply make you smile. Obviously, individual taste has a lot to do with what sorts of images work best. "Choose something that makes you feel relaxed and that you'd enjoy looking at every day," says Dr. Good.

Liven things up. If you can't always get out and enjoy the spectacle of nature, bring some of it in to you. Being around plants, flowers, and trees is therapeutic, says Busch. That's why more and more hospitals are adding "healing gardens," both indoors and out, for the benefit of their patients and their staffs. Putting some greenery in your office or home can stimulate a nurturing spirit and make you feel more at ease when you look at it.

Let There Be Light Therapy

For some people, a lack of light can be downright dangerous to their mental and phys-

How to Be Bright-Eyed

To maximize the power of sight, take care to keep your eyes sharp and healthy. Take a look at these tips.

Keep the shades down. Exposure to the sun's ultraviolet light puts you at risk for cataracts, so wear sunglasses with ultraviolet protection whenever you're driving or outside.

Eat for your eyes. Fruits and vegetables containing vitamins C and E and beta-carotene can slow cataract growth and promote eye health. For C, eat strawberries or cantaloupes. Almonds, peanut butter, and shrimp are high in E. And you'll find beta-carotene in white, yellow, and orange fruits and vegetables.

Get 'em checked. When was the last time you went to an eye doctor? If you have good vision and no history of problems, you ought to be going at least every three years.

ical health. During winter months, especially in the northern states where daylight tends to be scarce, some people experience greater-than-normal bouts of depression, fatigue, and lethargy.

The severity of these symptoms varies widely, according to Michael Terman, Ph.D., director of the winter depression program at the Columbia-Presbyterian Medical Center in New York City. Some people have what is called the winter blues or the winter doldrums, which is the relatively mild version that, in addition to a blue mood, involves intrusive bouts of fatigue, difficulty waking and feeling alert, and an increased appetite that centers around cravings for carbohydrate-rich foods. People with severe cases of these symptoms have seasonal affective disorder (SAD), and they qualify as seriously depressed. Estimates are that about 6 percent of the population can be diagnosed as having full-fledged SAD.

If you feel seriously depressed in the

winter and unable to keep up with your normal activities, you need to talk with your doctor to see if SAD has you down. But if you find that your milder symptoms just leave you feeling down at certain times, maybe what you need is to say to yourself, "Let there be light!" and follow this advice.

Take a walk. A daily 45-minute walk outside can help counteract seasonal depression. "Even when the sky is overcast, you're getting much more light than you do indoors," says Dr. Terman. "If possible, walk in the morning because the biological clock in your brain is more receptive to sunlight then. But even a lunchtime walk can have large benefits."

Light your way. Pay attention to how the indoor spaces where you spend time are lit, says Dr. Good. If you have windows, don't keep the blinds at half-mast. Crank them up. And if no window is available (as is often the case at work), turn on a couple extra lamps. Brightly lit spaces are generally more energetic, says Dr. Good. Dim lights, meanwhile, create a more womblike feeling. Natural lighting is best. Fluorescent lighting will give some people headaches from eyestrain.

Dr. Terman says that many older people with seasonal depression have a habit of leaving their lights off to save electricity. It's worth spending a few extra pennies a day to brighten your surroundings. Don't overdo it, though. Looking directly into a naked lightbulb, for example, can damage your eyes.

Equip yourself. If you want to get serious about it, you can buy a specially designed light box containing bright fluorescent lights and "dose" yourself with light for at least a half-hour every day, says Dr. Terman. The amount of time varies according to the type

Every Picture Tells a Story

We tend to think of artists as either nutcases or pansies: wild men who drink too much and cut their ears off, or overly sensitive types who sit around drawing daisies all day. Those stereotypes obscure the fact that art—drawing, painting, sculpture, even doodling—can help reveal what's really going on in our hearts and minds, showing us things we don't always allow ourselves to consciously see.

"You don't have to have any particular skill at art; you're not trying to win any prizes," says Linda Gantt, Ph.D., director of art therapy at the Trauma Recovery Institute in Morgantown, West Virginia, and past president of the American Art Therapy Association, which is headquartered in Mundelein, Illinois. "But when you put something on paper, it allows you to look at things in a different way—literally."

Here are some of Dr. Gantt's suggestions for getting a glimpse of yourself through art.

Set yourself up. Buy a sketch book or a pad of drawing paper and some markers or colored pencils (at least 12 colors). And get inexpensive paper; you don't want to feel constrained by working on the fancy stuff.

Let it flow. Each week, set aside a half-hour to an hour to draw, and pick a subject area that you want to focus on: your family, your work, your marriage, the future, maybe your childhood. Make drawings about how you feel about each particular subject. The more drawings, the better. Again, the point is expressing, freely and unself-consciously, your emotions. "See what kinds of lines, colors, and shapes you enjoy doing," says Dr. Gantt. "It doesn't have to be abstract, but don't feel that

of light fixture used and the individual using it, so check with your doctor for usage instructions based on your needs. Another form of treatment is called a dawn simulator, which is a light you have to do something realistic, either. Let your inner vision flow."

Are you having a hard time thinking of things to draw? Dr. Gantt often asks her patients to try drawing three wishes they would like to have come true. She also suggests trying to draw a depiction of the past, present, and the future; of roads not taken; or of the various masks you wear in different situations in your life.

Stand back. Once you have some images on paper, you can look at yourself from a new angle. Tape the pictures up on a wall and look at them from a distance, Dr. Gantt suggests. Cut a small hole in a piece of cardboard, then look at your pictures through the hole, from close up and from far away. Focus in on different parts of each picture. Put your drawings away and look at them a month later. With each viewing, you'll likely see a different part of yourself.

Look for clues. Try to see if any themes emerge in the drawings that give you clues about what's happening in your subconscious. Note any patterns you see in the shapes, the colors, and the relationships between the elements of your pictures. Do you use the color red a lot? Do jagged lines separate figures? Remember that the style and mood of a picture is often more significant than the specific subject matter. "It's not what the person draws," says Dr. Gantt, "but how he draws it."

Ultimately, nobody can be entirely certain what your pictures are saying—not even you. Think of them as hints that can start you thinking rather than as road maps that lead clearly to a specific destination.

light conditions. Research has shown that consistent exposure to extremely bright doses of fluorescent light can lessen or eliminate SAD symptoms in a substantial proportion of people who use it. Light boxes and dawn simulators are available from SunBox Company, 19217 Orbit Drive, Gaithersburg, MD 20879-4149.

The fixtures aren't cheap. A good light box can set you back $350 or more. For that reason, you may want to try a professional light therapy treatment before making the investment yourself. For a reference to a light therapist in your area, contact the Society for Light Treatment and Biological Rhythms, 10200 West 44th Avenue, Suite 304, Wheat Ridge, CO 80033-2840. There is a charge for member referrals. Be advised as well that no certification program for light therapists exists, so training and experience can vary substantially.

Watch for the signs. Some people have winter doldrums one year and then skip the next, Dr. Terman says. For that reason, he recommends that before you start light therapy, you wait until you sense that a depression is beginning to set in, unless you feel absolutely confident of your seasonal regularity. "If you know that this problem acts like clockwork, especially if it's very disturbing to you, go ahead and begin therapy a couple weeks before you expect the slump, so that you can nip it in the bud," he says.

On average, winter doldrums usually hit sometime in October, but the timing of their onset varies widely, Dr. Terman says. Some people start feeling blue in the late summer, and by February, they're beginning to feel better. Others don't start to sink until after New Year's. "You have to know your own cycle in order to use light therapy effectively," he says.

system installed over your bed that is programmed to go on in the early-morning hours, while you're still asleep. Both systems trick your brain into thinking you're actually in summer

The Power of Smell

Start Making Scents

It's hard to top the scent of a woman (to borrow a movie title), or of a new car, for that matter. But surely the smell of fresh sheets or the tantalizing odor of a neighborhood cookout ranks up there among life's more refreshing small pleasures. The pungent punch of eucalyptus and menthol in Vicks VapoRub is a very familiar healing odor. The smell of cedar is as much a part of a sauna as sweat is. Do you have any positive associations with the smell of a pinewood forest? Do you have any negative associations with the smell of a hospital? Ever had cinnamon on your cappuccino? Ever savored the scent of an after-dinner mint?

If you said yes to even one of the above questions, you already know how powerful your sense of smell is in triggering memories and stirring strong feelings. But what you smell can also play a role in your health and well-being, says Victoria Edwards, an aromatherapist in Fair Oaks, California. Aromatherapy tries to capitalize on the power of smell by using essential oils—distilled essences of various plants, trees, flowers, barks, and seeds—to calm, stimulate, and, supposedly, heal.

Some aromatherapists claim that essential oils are helpful in healing everything from burns to cancer, although little scientific research is available at this point to back that up. Studies on the health benefits of smell are hard to pin down because aroma is so, well, ineffable. Does a cer-

tain odor affect us because it stimulates a specific physiological process in our bodies, because it provokes certain psychological associations in our hearts, or both? We just don't know.

Despite these uncertainties, there's little question that aromas do have some effect on our moods and our behaviors. Studies have found, for example, that:

- When specific aromas were pumped into a test site in a casino, gamblers spent up to 53 percent more money at the slot machines.
- The smell of peppermint stimulated people to perform better on attention tests. The smell of lavender significantly slowed decision times, while the smell of jasmine increased them.
- When a scent resembling the smell of baby powder was circulated in a hospital examination room, patients experienced less anxiety.
- When fruity or floral scents were circulated in a jewelry store, people shopped longer. Pleasant scents also caused people to linger longer at museum exhibits.

Putting Smell to the Test

If you doubt that the power of aroma can tap into your own reservoir of memories and emotions, try taking a little three-step smell test of your own, suggests Edwards.

Step one: Gather together in a desk or dresser drawer a collection of aromatic objects that have scents you find pleasing and evocative. Individual choices may vary, but some good possibilities include:

- Your old baseball glove
- A can of Play-Doh
- A stick of cinnamon
- An after-dinner mint
- A stick of sandalwood incense

- Your wife or girlfriend's perfumed lingerie
- A container of baby powder

Step two: Now, give yourself a smell session. Close the door of your study or bedroom, draw the blinds, and sit down in a comfortable chair. Put on some soothing music if you like. Then, one by one, take out your aromatic objects and breathe deeply.

Step three: Close your eyes and free-associate. Relax. Do the smells take you to a different place? Do you find any of the smells inherently relaxing, comforting, or stimulating? Is there any corresponding change in your mood? Does it stimulate memories? That's the power of smell at work.

Putting Aroma to Work

Our little experiment in amateur aromatherapy can give a hint of the sorts of effects that true aromatherapy promises to achieve using far more refined and potent sources of smell. Professional aromatherapy is generally used in conjunction with other therapies—massage therapy, in particular—but it's one of the easiest alternative methods to use at home. Here are some guidelines for giving aromatherapy a try.

Buy a starter kit. Look for the colored vials of aromatherapy oils at your local health food store or New Age bookstore—heck, even the neighborhood gift shop likely has these oils in stock. Asked to choose a good beginner's selection of essential oils specifically for men, Edwards recommends these six scents: peppermint, lemon, eucalyptus, lavender, pine, and juniper. All have refreshing, soothing, and restorative qualities, she says. And all can be mixed and matched in various combinations.

Smells like Fun

Some alternative remedies can be a treat to try, and aphrodisiac aromas certainly would fit in that category. Here is a list of essential oils that aromatherapist Victoria Edwards thinks may have aphrodisiac qualities either because they help people relax or because they're sensually stimulating. Check with an aromatherapist about cautions and procedures before using these oils on your own.

Black pepper	Clove	Rose
Cardamom	Jasmine	Sandalwood
Cinnamon	Neroli	Ylang-ylang
Clary	Patchouli	

Edwards has compiled another list of oils that she believes can help overcome various types of emotional and psychological problems. Don't forget to check with an aromatherapist before using these.

Anger: chamomile, rosemary, ylang-ylang
Anxiety: bergamot, citrus oils, melissa
Depression: bergamot, clary, jasmine
Fear: geranium, hyssop, juniper
General stress: bergamot, geranium, lavender
Mental stress: basil, citrus oils, lemongrass, neroli, sandalwood

Part of the fun of aromatherapy is coming up with blends of oils that suit you personally. Because some essential oils can irritate people with sensitive skin, it is best to talk to a professional aromatherapist to find which oils are right for you.

Other scents that men gravitate toward, Edwards says, include clary, fir, and cedar, while lavender and spikenard tend to appeal equally to both men and women.

Be safe. Some methods for diffusing aromas into the air can be hazardous to your health. Burning incense is one of them; research has shown that incense smoke is a carcinogen, according to Edwards.

Putting the oil directly onto a lightbulb is even more dangerous. In theory, the heat of the bulb will disperse the oil through the room. In practice, the oil can cause the lightbulb to explode; or it can drip into the light fixture, causing a short. Dropping the oil on a candle or in candle wax is also risky. "Essential oils are highly volatile, which means that they're highly flammable," says aromatherapist and herbalist Jeanne Rose, executive director of the Aromatic Plant Project, a nonprofit organization based in San Francisco, and author of *The World of Aromatherapy.* "If you want to start a lovely fire, you can use essential oils as lighter fluid."

Don't drink it in. Although it's perfectly safe to inhale the scent of aromatherapy oils, only very small amounts are therapeutic and should be used only upon the advice of a trained, professional aromatherapist. Never drink essential oils, says Edwards.

Breathe it in. Companies sell lots of different types of equipment for diffusing essential oils into the air you breathe, but you don't need any of them. "Put three or four drops on a cotton ball, a tissue, or a handkerchief, and hold it up to your nose," says Edwards. Take a sniff or two and repeat as often as you like.

For a more direct approach, Edwards recommends adding five to eight drops of essential oil to a bowl of steaming water. Place a towel over both your head and the bowl and inhale the vapor for a few minutes. Be careful that the water is not too hot and that you don't get close enough to it to burn your face.

Rub it in. One of the more enjoyable ways to experience aromatherapy is to have a massage with aromatically scented oil, either by yourself or with your partner. For a single massage, Edwards suggests that you fill a saucer with about an ounce of unscented massage oil and

Keep Your Nose Healthy

If you want to take advantage of the power of smell, you'll need to make sure that your sniffer stays up to snuff. Here are some quick tips for good nasal health.

Avoid allergens. Chronic sinus infections and allergies account for one-quarter of the cases of smell loss. If you suffer from allergies but don't know what you're allergic to, get tested.

Go easy on the antihistamines. Although they'll unstuff a clogged nose, antihistamines and decongestants can dry out the nose too much. Instead, use a nasal spray to decongest. This will also keep your nose moist. And, as your dog could tell you, a moist nose is a healthy nose.

See red and yellow. Fruits and vegetables in these hues are high in vitamin A, which helps maintain a healthy nasal lining.

mix into it 10 to 20 drops of essential oil. Although many essential oils can be beneficial for the skin, they are highly concentrated and, therefore, should never be applied at full strength.

Soak it in. Soaking in a scented bath isn't considered a manly thing, but if you have a lock on the bathroom door, you owe it to yourself to try it. Simply run a warm bath, add five to eight drops of essential oil mixed with about an ounce of milk, and hop in, says Edwards.

Drive it home. One of the most stressful places you can possibly be is on a crowded city highway at rush hour. Edwards recommends turning your car into an "aromamobile" by putting a few drops of essential oil on a paper towel or a cloth and setting it on the dashboard. The heat from the sun or the car heater will help diffuse the oil, she says. Add some soft music and you'll have a more restful commute, even in traffic.

The Power of Hearing

Sounds Good to Us

In the movie *Stand by Me*, four boys set out on a quest that takes them through dense, dark forests and leech-infested swamps. They've lied to their parents about what they're doing; they have a long way to go. They're excited, but also scared. To ward off the heebie-jeebies, they start singing the theme song from the 1950s TV show *Have Gun Will Travel*.

Little did this fictional band of kids know that they had initiated a spontaneous session of music therapy, employing a familiar song at an anxious moment to provide some communal reassurance and to gain inner strength by identifying with something more powerful than themselves. Music—or even just soothing sounds—has been used in just that way throughout human history to help us cope with everything from facing down fearsome beasts in the jungle to approaching fearsome females in singles bars. Indeed, music's powers of courage, comfort, and inspiration are so accessible that many of us in the modern world tend to take them for granted.

Part of the reason that music and sounds are such potent forces is that they effortlessly bridge mind, body, and spirit. The sounds we hear have a direct impact on the limbic system of the brain, the seat of emotions and a gateway to memory, which helps explain why Miles, Muddy, or Mozart can so powerfully move us; why we tend to associate first kisses and first jobs with the songs that were playing when we experienced them; and why the phrase "whistling past the graveyard" carries any meaning at all in our society.

Making Music Work

The exact mechanisms of how music's emotional and physical effects interact with one another is still largely a mystery, but there's no doubt that their combination can have an impact on health. Thousands of music therapists are hard at work in hospitals, schools, and rehabilitation centers across the country, using music to treat everything from attention deficit disorder to Alzheimer's disease. Outside the hospitals, music and soothing sounds can be key forms of psychic self-defense against two of the biggest hazards of modern life: stress and depression.

Listening to music and making music can change our moods much like drugs can, says Paul Nolan, a certified music therapist and director of music therapy education at Allegheny University of the Health Sciences in Philadelphia. "What that means is that we all have our own music medicine chest with us all the time."

Here are some ways you can most effectively put the power of music to use in your life.

Schedule a music meditation. Music is an extremely effective focus for meditation, whether you're a monk in a monastery or an atheist in a hotel room. Set aside 20 to 30 minutes at a time of the day when you can afford to relax, Nolan says, and find a place where you will be able to focus your attention completely on the music. "Most of us use music as background noise while we're doing something else," he says. "The point of this exercise is to make the music a primary source of stimulation, not an accessory."

Nolan recommends sitting in a comfortable chair or lying down and "thinking the music," by which he means listening carefully to what the instruments are doing, both individually and in concert with each other. Pay attention to what's happening in the background as well as the foreground of the piece. If you find yourself thinking about something other than the music, redirect those thoughts. Tell yourself that you'll think about that later. Then bring your attention back to the music.

Shop for sounds. What kind of music works best for meditation? "Look for music that slows down your heart rate," says Steven Halpern, Ph.D., president of Inner Peace Music in San Anselmo, California, and a composer. "If you play slow music, your heartbeat will slow down. Fast music will speed it up. The phenomenon known as rhythm entrainment is an involuntary response to an external rhythmic stimulus. Your heartbeat literally will march to the beat of a different drummer."

Dr. Halpern also recommends music that is not overly "busy." "When it comes to relaxation, sometimes less is more," he says. The body is not necessarily impressed by complexity. Complex music is like a big meal; it's hard to digest. Better choices might be certain classical pieces—especially the slow movements in symphonies and concertos.

Build a library. Once you find a selection of mood music that suits you, take it along when you travel, suggests Michael Rohrbacher, Ph.D., a certified music therapist and director of music therapy at Shenandoah University in Winchester, Virginia. The power of association can help rekindle a relaxed state of mind as soon as you hear it, wherever you might be.

Seek what soothes. Music doesn't have to enhance meditation to make us feel better. We can derive great psychological comfort from songs and musical styles that are associated with our personal experiences. That means that different people can have quite different responses to the same type of music. A colleague of Nolan's told him about a fright-

ened 16-year-old being wheeled into surgery who was instantly calmed when a song by the rock band Nine Inch Nails came blasting through his headphones. Played for his grandfather, the same song would likely have killed the man. "The style of music that I like best is custom tailored for me, by me, over a lifetime of listening. And my neurology is going to respond to that immediately," Nolan says.

Play an instrument. Beating on an instrument is a form of exercise, Dr. Halpern points out, which enhances everything from the production of endorphins to the supply of oxygen in the brain. Playing music can also be a simple, virtually automatic form of meditation. "If you're making music," Dr. Halpern says, "you can't be doing something else." So if you haven't picked up that guitar or sax in years, break it out and tune it up—and get yourself in tune.

Sound a gong. If you don't play an instrument, try using a simple rhythmic instrument like a drum. Drumming can be an especially effective way to break free of that driving pace, because it directly creates a new vibration to which your body can adjust. "Drumming is a great way to cleanse the psychological system," says Don Campbell, a music therapist who lectures on the healthful benefits of music, director of the Mozart Effect Resource Center in St. Louis, and author of *The Mozart Effect: Tapping the Power of Music to Heal the Body, Strengthen the Mind, and Unlock the Creative Spirit.* "Ten minutes of drumming every day releases tension and resets the mind and the body's inner clock."

Campbell recommends sitting comfortably in a chair with anything that you can make a sound with—a plastic wastebasket and a couple of sticks works just as well as a drum set, he says. Close your eyes and listen for your heartbeat, then start beating in time with it. After a few minutes, try to double the beat so that it's twice as fast as your heart. After three minutes of that, return to a beat that matches your basic heartbeat and notice whether it has become faster or slower. Then reduce the number of your drumbeats to match every other beat of your heart.

Campbell stresses that you don't need a keenly developed sense of rhythm to try this exercise. "You cannot make a mistake," he says, "as long as you're not too loud."

Drum some sense into the world. When you've had an especially crazy day, you can try a two-stage drumming exercise that will help you regain your composure, says Dr. Rohrbacher. In the first stage, simply let it all hang out: Direct your passions into the drum, or whatever you're using as a drum, gradually building up the intensity of your pounding as far as you can let it go, to the point of complete frenzy and chaos. In the second stage, build your rhythm up again, but just before you reach the crescendo, consciously lower the level of intensity a bit and channel your beat into a more structured, steadier rhythm. Begin chanting along with your drumming, if you like. Move from repeated expressions such as "I'm so damn angry!" to "I can get through this!" and finally to "Yes! . . . Yes!"—whatever suits the situation.

What you're doing as you take this musical journey, Dr. Rohrbacher says, is demonstrating to yourself than you can consciously impose a meaningful structure on a world that appears to be out of your control. "It's a very safe place to put your anger," he says, "a much better one than threatening to hit someone or throwing a chair against the wall."

Join a jam. Playing music with others is healthier still. Numerous studies have shown that social interaction can help ward off disease, and the relationship you have with others when you're jamming—backing one another up during solos, striving to blend your efforts harmoniously, even helping carry equipment be-

White Noise Addiction

We don't have to tell you how noisy the modern world has become. All that racket isn't healthy, psychologically or physically. The question is, what can you do about it?

One solution is to create some relatively benign sounds of your own, sounds that will mask and neutralize the unwanted intrusive noises that civilization throws your way. Such sounds are called white noise. Dentists use a form of white noise when they put on soft rock to mask the grinding sound of their drills. White noise machines have become a common household appliance. Turn them on and they fill your bedroom or office with the soothing sounds of wind, waves, or rainstorms—although some say that the sound is more like radio static.

The problem with using white noise as a long-term solution, according to Paul Nolan of Allegheny University of the Health Sciences, is that it can become habit-forming. "A friend of mine conditioned himself to sleeping with a white noise machine," he says. "Now he has to take it with him whenever he travels, because he can't sleep in hotels without it." If you're going to use white noise to help you sleep or calm down, it may be best to use it only once in awhile, he adds.

fore and after a session—epitomizes constructive, cooperative social interaction. "You have the feeling of being involved with something greater than yourself," says Nolan. "You're collaborating on a common goal, which is producing something of beauty."

This doesn't mean that you need any talent to enjoy the benefits of musical bonding, Nolan quickly adds. Bonding is the point.

The Power of Food

Eating Your Way toward Health

Fact: Diet contributes to 4 of the top 10 causes of death per year in the United States. Experts estimate that we could save more than $23 billion a year on hospitalization costs alone if Americans took on a more healthy diet.

But food doesn't just play a part in your death; it greatly impacts your quality of life. Other chronic diseases related to diet—cataracts, memory loss, diabetes, obesity, high blood pressure, impaired immune function—might not kill you directly, but they sure won't make life more enjoyable.

View food as more than fuel. View food as a potent healing agent and disease-fighter. If you do, you might be pleasantly surprised at how quickly your meal choices can lead to a better, stronger, healthier you, not just in the long term but day to day as well. It's true: What you put in your mouth this morning can determine how you act, feel, and perform all day. "The right and wrong foods affect energy levels, weight gain, performance—things that a lot of guys actually care about," says Neal Barnard, M.D., president of the Physicians Committee for Responsible Medicine in Washington, D.C., and author of *Foods That Fight Pain.*

Often Imitated, Never Duplicated

Despite man's understanding of the world and our ability to create works of ad-

vanced technology, nature still humbles us with its simple power to pack a complex array of disease-fighting, life-sustaining substances into foodstuffs. We're talking about vitamins and minerals, sure, but also the newer world of antioxidants and flavonoids, part of a class of ingredients known as phytochemicals. These chemicals, which can only be found in plant foods, may fight all kinds of diseases, including heart disease and cancer, says Robert Cullen, R.D., Ph.D., assistant professor of food and nutrition, and nutrition and dietetics program director at Illinois State University in Normal.

But don't expect these phytochemicals to make an appearance in your multivitamin anytime soon. Unlike the limited number of vitamins and minerals, there are thousands of phytochemicals, and researchers aren't entirely clear what they do or how they work, either separately or together. To get the potential health benefits of these chemicals, you can't pop a pill. You have to go to the source.

"The most natural way to get the nutrients and phytochemicals that you need is in food," says Maria G. Boosalis, R.D., Ph.D., associate professor in the division of clinical nutrition in the College of Allied Health Professions at the University of Kentucky in Lexington. Indeed, as far as phytochemicals are concerned, it's the only way.

The Big Three

Primitive man may have lived a nasty, brutish, and short life, but he had one factor in his favor: he knew how to eat. He relied on fruits, vegetables, and grains and only dabbled in eating meat and other fattening foods, says Gene Spiller, Ph.D., a nutrition researcher, director of the Health Research and Studies Center in Los Altos, California, and co-author of *Nutrition Secrets of the Ancients.* So should you. Here's why.

Fruits and vegetables. Study after study links a diet high in fruits and vegetables to lower cancer rates, less incidence of heart disease, prevention of disease of the blood vessels around the brain, and reduced blood pressure. Despite this overwhelming evidence, only 22 percent of Americans eat the recommended five or more servings a day.

To gain the full health benefits of fruits and vegetables, you have to become a man of varied tastes. Eating five bananas each day won't do you much good. Each fruit and vegetable has its own stable of disease-preventing powerhouses. "While many fruits and vegetables have these different chemicals, no single one has them all. You need variety," says Laurie Meyer, R.D., a nutritionist in private practice in Milwaukee.

But the tomato should hold a special place in the hearts and prostates of men. A study at Harvard showed that men who ate two or more servings of tomato products a week reduced their risks of prostate cancer by as much as 34 percent. And tomato sauce, not just the tomato, gave the greatest protective benefit. So go ahead and call your local pizza pie man. Tell him to go heavy on the sauce, easy on the cheese and pepperoni.

High-fiber diet. First, soluble fiber, found in foods like certain whole-grain cereals and breads, apples (and other fruits), and beans (as well as other legumes) reduces your body's levels of artery-hardening cholesterol and by-products of cholesterol by soaking them up and carrying them out of your digestive system. Meanwhile, insoluble fiber—undigestible roughage found in the skins of fruits

No Need to Sneak Snacks

Just like any other food choice you make, snacks can help or hurt your overall health. You can turn your midday or late-night cravings into a health-enhancing exercise—and you don't have to munch on wood pulp to do it. Here are some healthy yet satisfying snack ideas.

- Fill your desk drawer with instant soups. "Noodle soups sound like they're just for kids, but they're a great snack for everybody," says Dr. Neal Barnard of the Physicians Committee for Responsible Medicine. Stock up on vegetarian soups with fiber-rich lentils.

- Grab an orange or an apple when you feel the hunger pangs. If you travel a lot and get the munchies while driving, keep a cooler with fruit in the backseat, says Melanie R. Polk, R.D., director of nutrition education at the American Institute for Cancer Research in Washington, D.C.

- Go easy on the chips and heavy on the salsa. Each swipe of salsa contains antioxidants, phytochemicals, and many other needed substances found in fruits and vegetables. "Salsa is a nice way of getting fruits and vegetables in your diet without even thinking about it," says nutritionist Laurie Meyer.

- A snack of dried fruit and nuts can match the strongest sugar and salt cravings. Keep a box of raisins, prunes, or figs around and mix them with a handful of nuts, recommends Dr. Gene Spiller of the Health Research and Studies Center.

and vegetables (potatoes and apples are classic examples) as well as in whole-grain products—absorbs water, and bulks up stool and speeds its movement out of the body, carrying disease-causing particles with it.

Fiber may also be able to help you to shed some pounds or keep the weight off. Fiber slows down your digestion process, making you feel full longer and less likely to chow down. In a study conducted at the University of Leeds in the United Kingdom, 16 men were given breakfasts containing either soluble or insoluble fiber. The insoluble fiber group felt fuller after breakfast, while the soluble fiber group reported feeling satisfied well into the day. A diet high in both fibers may help curb your appetite all day long.

Low-fat diet. That cheese steak with french fries may taste good going down, but soon after it hits your stomach, it starts pumping up your cholesterol levels. Keep those cholesterol levels high enough, and over time, your arteries start to clog up, restricting blood to your brain, your heart, and that other vital organ, your penis. While the amount of blood pulsing around starts to decrease, your waistline will start to do the opposite.

The American Heart Association recommends reducing dietary fat to 30 percent of your total calories. Just by cutting down to 30 percent, you can decrease your total cholesterol level anywhere from 10 to 20 percent, which puts you at lower risk for life-threatening problems like heart disease and stroke.

But fat isn't always your sworn enemy. A certain kind of fat—monounsaturated fat—may actually help your health. Monounsaturated fats may raise or maintain your good high-density lipoprotein (HDL) cholesterol, found in olive and canola oil. The HDL cholesterol keeps the "bad" low-density lipoprotein (LDL) cholesterol from clogging up your arteries. By using monounsaturated fats, you can lower the number of bad guys in your bloodstream while raising the number of good guys.

A study in Australia found that a low-fat diet supplemented with the monounsaturated fat–rich olive oil was healthier than an extremely low fat diet without the olive oil. Both diets lowered the total and LDL cholesterol levels. But only the olive oil diet kept the HDL levels from dropping. To get the benefits of monounsaturated fats, use olive oil and canola oil when cooking. That's not to say that you can go nuts with oil. Fats still shouldn't be more than 30 percent of your total calories, says Dr. Spiller.

By the way, meat-lovers, cutting back on fat doesn't mean that you have to become a vegetarian. You just have to make leaner choices. Stick to leaner meats such as top round, bottom round, and sirloin tip, and limit yourself to three ounces a day—about the size of a deck of cards or the palm of your hand, Meyer says.

Putting It into Practice

On paper, eating a healthy, mostly plant-based diet makes all the sense in the world. But putting that theory into practice may seem a little daunting, says Melanie R. Polk of the American Institute for Cancer Research.

Contrary to what you might think, eating healthy doesn't mean a major change in your lifestyle; nor do your tastebuds have to suffer. Small changes—adding some fruits and vegetables here, trimming some fat there—is all you really need. As you'll see, changing your diet for the better will only take a little tweaking. Here are some tips to get you started.

Shopping

Stock up the pantry. The fast-food joint down on the corner looks irresistible when you open your kitchen cabinet to find cartons of food dating back to the previous presidential administration. If you keep a reserve of certain ingredients in your kitchen at all times, you can make a simple and healthy meal within minutes, says Polk. Items that should always be on hand include canned fruit in juices; canned tomatoes; whole-grain pasta; a bag of brown rice; assorted beans; low-fat chicken broth; a variety of sauces, including low-fat tomato, soy, barbecue, and teriyaki sauces; flavored vinegars; cooking wine; cornstarch; and honey. You will find more items to stock in the following tips.

Find the frozen tundra. The frozen-food aisle in the supermarket holds more than waffles and ice cream. It is a mecca of vegetables. Frozen vegetables have just as much nutrition—if not more—than fresh, Polk says. Search for medleys that offer up to five and six different kinds of vegetables. Make them as a side dish, or toss them into pasta dishes, soups, and stir-fry meals. Other items to keep in the freezer include chicken breasts and whole-grain breads. Thanks to the defrost setting on the microwave, you can have meals ready to go in no time.

Buy seasonal and long-lived fruits. You should buy a variety of fresh fruits often so that you can benefit from the multitude of nutrients and phytochemicals. Especially stock up on apples and oranges, Polk says. Left in the refrigerator, these fruits keep for weeks. Buy a bunch of both so that you are always sure to have fruit on hand.

White out white breads and rice. To get more fiber into your diet without even thinking about it, purchase whole-grain breads, crackers, cereals, and brown rice. All contain more fiber than their refined counterparts, which have been stripped of the fiber-rich part of the grain. The words *whole grain* should be the first in the ingredients list, Polk says.

Stick to low-fat fare. Although milk, cheeses, and many other dairy products can be healthy sources of vitamins and minerals like calcium, the fat they contain can add up over time. Save yourself some fat grams by buying low-fat or skim milk, and low-fat cheeses and yogurts, Meyer says.

Making Meals

Hit the sauce. Guys especially should go heavy using salsa, tomato sauce, and canned tomatoes. Tomato products contain the phytochemical lycopene, which has been shown to cut the risk of prostate cancer, Meyer says. A quick dinner of pasta and tomato sauce with low-fat chips and salsa as a second course is not only healthy but also easy to prepare.

In One Swift Stroke

Making one change—just one simple change—to your diet could knock out a bevy of diseases. Unlike pills, which are limited to treating a specific problem, food covers a lot more ground. For example, you may want to cut out some fat in your diet to prevent heart disease. But by doing so, you also decrease your chances of developing cancer, diabetes, obesity, and cataracts.

Here are three changes you can make to your diet and the positive and preventive effects they will have on a variety of diseases.

	Decrease Fat	Increase Antioxidants	Increase Fiber
Helps prevent heart disease	x	x	x
Helps prevent cancer	x	x	x
Helps prevent diabetes	x	x	x
Helps prevent obesity	x		x
Helps prevent cataracts	x	x	
Bolsters immune function	x	x	x

Pile it on. Even a basic sandwich has room for more servings of vegetables. Use a piece or two of lean meat and low-fat cheese, but stuff the bread with dark green lettuce, tomatoes, and onions, Meyer says.

Make meat a minority. Meat doesn't have to disappear from your menu; just make it a supporting actor. Vegetables, whole grains, and beans should take up at least half your plate. "Meat should be considered a condiment to the vegetables," Dr. Spiller says.

Search for alternatives. Love tacos? Try them with chicken or beans. Got a craving for some chili? Throw in some turkey instead of beef. "You don't have to get rid of meat, but try to use more fish and skinless poultry," Meyer says. Chicken, beans, turkey, and fish give you the meaty feel without the fat. If you really want to try something new, search for ostrich or buffalo meat. "It tastes like beef but has the fat content of chicken," Meyer says.

Slip yourself some skin. Fruit and vegetable skins usually house the majority of the fiber. By peeling an apple or discarding a potato skin, you lose a vital part of its benefits. If the skin is edible, eat it, Dr. Cullen says. When eating oranges and grapefruit, peel the skin instead of cutting the fruit into pieces. Peeling keeps more of the white stringy membrane on the fruit. The white membrane contains pectin, the soluble fiber linked to lowering cholesterol.

Soak up some spice. By adding a little bit of flavoring to meats and vegetables, you can enhance the taste without adding fat, Meyer says. Season vegetables and meats with herbs and spices. Cook with flavored vinegars and sauces like soy and teriyaki. Use low-fat salad dressing as a meat marinade.

Fire up the grill. Eating plain steamed broccoli day in and day out would drive a lot of people into the arms of french fries. But eating vegetables doesn't have to be that way. Just a little culinary tinkering greatly improves the tongue-tingling effect of vegetables. Marinate the vegetables in a little bit of olive oil or soy sauce and throw them on the grill. "They are wonderful that way," Meyer says. Or mix a cup of low-fat chicken broth with one to two tablespoons of olive oil and glaze peppers, potatoes, mushrooms, and squash (or any vegetable mix you like). Roast them in the oven for about a half-hour.

Make your own pizza. Instead of calling up the local pizza joint, whip up your own pizza pie. Just grab a premade pizza crust and top it with low-fat tomato sauce, low-fat mozzarella cheese, pieces of cooked chicken, and a slew of vegetables, Meyer says. Stick it into the oven and bake for as long as the directions recommend. You get an easy, tasty dinner that is loaded with disease-fighting compounds at the same time. And you don't have to tip the delivery boy.

Eating Out

Travel the world. "It pays to think ethnic when eating out," Dr. Barnard says. International fare offers tasty low-fat dishes that stress fruits, vegetables, grains, and beans. Get the spaghetti marinara at the Italian restaurant, a bean burrito at a Mexican place, or a vegetable stir-fry at a Chinese takeout.

Head to the bars. Many supermarkets and even fast-food places now offer salad and baked potato bars. "And they are good, too. It's not just lettuce anymore," Dr. Barnard says. Load up on the various vegetables and even legumes such as chickpeas, he says. Make sure that you have lots of colors on your plate. Add a little low-fat salad dressing or vinegar and you are good to go. Cover your baked potato with veggies as well, instead of opting for fat-laden butter and sour cream.

Use the one-for-two special. If you're eating at a deli or a restaurant that believes that a portion size should feed a small country, split one meal between you and a friend. "If it is a giant-size sandwich, cut it in half and share it," Polk says.

Experiment. When eating out, order all kinds of vegetables prepared in all different types of ways—things that you'd never think of at home. Decide what you like (and what you don't), and then incorporate them into you meals at home, Dr. Barnard says.

Making a Meal Plan

Once you've stocked up the pantry, it's time to test your skills at home. You have an endless variety of meals to choose from that taste great while tapping the power of food. Dr. Barnard recommends the following sample meal plan to get you started. Feel free to add, subtract, and generally get creative with it.

Breakfast

Pick a high-fiber cereal and top it with bananas, strawberries, or blueberries. If you don't care for the taste of high-fiber cereals, mix one with a cereal you do like. Use low-fat (1%) or skim milk for your cereal. Drink an eight-ounce glass of orange juice.

Or have a bowl of oatmeal made with low-fat (1%) or skim milk. Top the oatmeal with fruit and ground cinnamon to add flavor. Add a piece of whole-wheat toast covered with fruit jam and a few slices of melon. Drink an eight-ounce glass of orange juice.

Or make pancakes but add a half-cup of wheat germ to the batter to increase the fiber. Top pancakes with bananas or strawberries. Drink an eight-ounce glass of orange juice.

Lunch

Put a veggie burger on two slices of whole-wheat bread. Top the sandwich with dark green lettuce, onions, and tomatoes, and add mustard or low-fat mayonnaise. Eat an apple or an orange for dessert.

Or try a bean burrito topped with salsa, low-fat cheese, lettuce, and tomato. Have a salad with low-fat or fat-free dressing. Load up on dark greens and red and orange vegetables and top with low-fat salad dressing. Eat a slice of whole-grain bread or a dinner roll. Have a fruit salad as dessert.

Dinner

Have some bean chili and a green salad. Also, grill up some vegetables such as zucchini or squash, peppers, or mushrooms marinated in a little olive oil. Serve with a side of quick-cooking brown rice.

Dissecting the Diets

You have alternative music, alternative medicine, even alternative diets. These left-of-mainstream diets range from not eating anything at all to eating only fruits and vegetables. Keep in mind that if you decide to make any major changes in your diet, you should always check with your doctor first.

Fasting. Fasting is refraining from food while your nutritional reserves are high enough to sustain your normal functions. As soon as those reserves hit zero, you begin starving. You need to break the fast before your body starts digging into vital tissues for its energy.

Detox diet. Detoxification involves dietary and lifestyle changes that reduce the intake of toxins and improve elimination. To eliminate these toxins, you avoid chemicals (from food or other sources), refined food, sugar, caffeine, alcohol, and tobacco and rely on water, fruits and vegetables, and grains for up to three weeks.

Raw foods diet. You eat only raw fruits, vegetables, nuts, seeds, and sprouts: fresh, whole, and unprocessed.

Macrobiotic diet. Based on traditional Oriental medicine, a macrobiotic diet is 50 to 60 percent whole grains, 20 to 25 percent vegetables, 5 to 10 percent seaweeds and beans, and 5 to 10 percent soups every day.

Elimination diet. People go on elimination diets when they suspect that they have food allergies. You eliminate the suspected food from your diet for several weeks, after which you eat it. If allergic symptoms reappear, you probably have an allergy to that food.

Or cook up some whole-wheat pasta and add a package of mixed frozen vegetables. Cover with low-fat tomato sauce. Add some garlic and fresh parsley for extra flavor.

The Power of Drink

The Healing Cup Overflows

You could survive for weeks without food, but you would only last for a few days without fluids. Without enough to drink, bodily functions would cease to work. But while drinking enough can keep you alive, drinking the right stuff can help you thrive. Some beverages contain cancer-fighting and heart disease–fighting compounds that many foods can't even touch.

Tea for Two Reasons

Drinking tea may evoke images of English gentility fussing about with china cups and platters of crumpets. But tea is anything but gentle when it comes to battling two major health hazards for men—heart disease and cancer. "Tea has all the positives, and it doesn't have any negatives," says Joe A. Vinson, Ph.D., professor of chemistry at the University of Scranton in Pennsylvania.

Tea contains compounds called polyphenols. Some of the most powerful polyphenols are known as flavonoids. These compounds act as antioxidants in your body, meaning that they neutralize unstable molecules called free radicals, Dr. Vinson says. It's these free radicals that roam around your body causing the damage that eventually leads to cancer and heart disease.

Herbal teas aren't really teas, by the way. Real tea comes from the warm-weather evergreen tree known as *Camellia sinensis.* Look for the word *tea* in the ingredients list or make sure that it doesn't say *herbal.* Here's a sampling of different kinds of health-enhancing teas.

Black tea. The tea bags you buy at your local supermarket contain black tea, which has powerful health benefits. Researchers have found that black tea helps keep low-density lipoprotein (LDL, the "bad") cholesterol from oxidizing, and this lowers your risk of heart disease.

Green tea. Both black tea and green tea have established themselves as cancer-fighters, says John H. Weisburger, M.D., Ph.D., senior member of the American Health Foundation in Valhalla, New York. Various studies have linked green tea with decreased rates of esophageal cancer, colon cancer, rectal cancer, and pancreatic cancer. Look for it at most health food stores and in some supermarkets.

Iced tea. If you make iced tea the old-fashioned way—brewing it yourself using tea bags—you'll get the same amount of the disease-fighting compounds as you would if you drank hot tea, Dr. Weisburger says. To make a quart of iced tea, pour a pint of hot water over four tea bags. Let it steep for five minutes, and then pour the tea concentrate in a quart-size container full of ice.

A Toast to Your Health

Back in 1982, researchers at the American Cancer Society asked 490,000 men and women ranging in age from 30 to 104 about their alcohol habits and then tracked their health over the next nine years. The findings showed that those who drank one alcoholic drink a day had 21 percent lower death rates from all causes than nondrinkers had. Those who imbibed also had 30 to 40 percent lower death rates from heart disease. People who had high risks of heart disease or stroke benefited the most from a drink a day, says Michael J. Thun, M.D., study author and director of analytic epidemiology at the American Cancer Society in Atlanta.

But you have to read the small print—just *one* drink daily. That's a 12-ounce beer, 5 ounces of wine, or 1½ ounces of 80-proof distilled spirits. As soon as you drink more than one, your death risk starts to swell. "Nothing in excess; moderation is the point," Dr. Thun says.

Certain alcohol beverages contain an extra-healthy kick to them. So if you are going to knock one down, get some additional benefit by making it one of the following.

Beer. Dark beer is rich in flavonoids, which may help prevent clots from forming along artery walls, a process that leads to heart attacks or strokes. If dark beer is a bit too heavy for you, take heart: Any kind of beer may help your ticker. One review of the scientific literature by American and European doctors found that there is substantial evidence that consuming moderate amounts of any alcoholic drink, including beer, is linked with a lower risk of heart disease.

Red wine. Red wine also contains the flavonoids that are found in dark beer and tea, Dr. Vinson says. Researchers in Israel found that drinking moderate amounts of red wine can help to slow the oxidation of LDL cholesterol, the process that causes heart disease.

Jumping for Juices

Nutrition experts recommend getting at least five servings of fruits and vegetables a day as part of a healthy lifestyle. If this seems a little daunting to you, relax. Disease-fighting vita-

> # Water, Water Everywhere
> **Drink eight, eight-ounce glasses of water a day. If you have to ask why, here's a quick reminder of the healing powers of nature's most basic nutrient.**
> - **Increases endurance during exercise**
> - **Lessens the effect of jet lag**
> - **Prevents and fights constipation**
> - **Lowers risk of developing kidney stones**
> - **Helps you lose weight**

mins, minerals, nutrients, and antioxidants can all be found in a nice tall glass of juice.

A lot of products called juice really contain mostly sugar, water, dye, preservatives—and maybe a little bit of juice. Buy as close to 100 percent juice as possible. Also, look for "purchase by" dates so that you get the freshest juice available. The fresher the juice, the more nutrients you get, says Eve Campanelli, Ph.D., a holistic family practitioner in private practice in Beverly Hills, California. A few juices stand out for special health conditions.

Grape juice. Grape juice is the nondrinker's red wine, Dr. Vinson says. Drink it to help ward off cancer and heart disease.

Tomato juice. A study at Harvard showed that men who ate two or more servings of tomato products a week significantly reduced their risks of prostate cancer. Tomato juice contains lycopene, an antioxidant linked to preventing prostate cancer, says Dr. Gene Spiller of the Health Research and Studies Center.

Pineapple juice. Dr. Campanelli says that pineapple juice is good for colds. The vitamin C in it helps clean out mucous membranes. But pineapple juice also may take the bite out of swelling. Pineapple contains an enzyme called bromelain, which has anti-inflammatory properties. It may also help with bursitis and tendinitis.

The Power of Herbs

*A Growing Field
of Natural Choices*

It used to be that you had to roam the wild forests of the Amazon or—just as taxing—navigate your way through the local health food store in order to partake of herbal healing. Now, you can find herbal teas, tinctures, and capsules while cruising down the aisles at many supermarkets.

Herbs keep edging their way into the mainstream of medical treatment. In a study by a supplement company, researchers found that 23 percent of the population uses herbal remedies—11 percent on a regular basis and the other 12 percent for specific conditions. To cap off the idea that herbs are a booming and lucrative business, over-the-counter pharmaceutical giants such as SmithKline Beecham and Warner-Lambert have jumped into the herbal supplement market.

What does this herbal bumper crop mean for you? More options. And with more options comes more power over your health. With herbs, you have natural and safer ways of preventing, or aiding the healing of, many diseases without relying on prescription drugs. After all, herbs are the natural forefathers of all the medications we have today. "They're what Mother Nature gave us. Herbs work, and they don't have all the side effects," says holistic family practitioner Dr. Eve Campanelli.

An Herbal Hand Guide

With the onslaught of herbal products clamoring for attention on the shelves, you may find yourself a little intimidated when trying to figure out what products to buy. Here are some general pointers about buying and taking herbs.

Buy standardized products whenever you can. Standardized means that the herbs have been processed to guarantee a known minimum level of one or more of the active ingredients. With these products, you'll know exactly how much of the active ingredients you are getting.

Buy them as fresh as possible. Some herbs have a short shelf life. Ask store personnel how long the product has been sitting out, says Dr. Campanelli.

Follow the directions. Each company may put different amounts of the active ingredient in its teas, tinctures, or pills. That's why one product label may tell you to take three pills twice a day, while another may tell you to take only a pill a day, says acupuncturist Victor S. Sierpina, M.D., assistant professor of family medicine at the University of Texas Medical Branch in Galveston. So follow instructions carefully.

Be patient. Because conventional pharmaceuticals are often highly concentrated forms of an herbal ingredient, you may not see the same quick results with herbs that you do with modern drugs, Dr. Sierpina says. While it might take longer than you're used to, you may also have fewer side effects than you would from taking a more powerful, synthetic form of the same active ingredient.

Watch for side effects. That said, don't assume that you can take more than the recommended doses just because herbs are natural. They can have side effects, too,

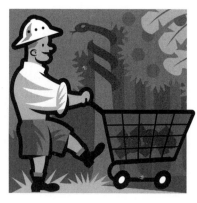

and can interact with other drugs you might be taking. If you are taking any prescription drugs, check with your doctor before taking any herbs, recommends Dr. Sierpina. Read labels carefully for noted side effects. If you experience any, stop taking the remedy.

Herbs Making Headlines

While all kinds of herbal remedies have increased in popularity, a few special herbs have been thrust out into the spotlight. Here's a list of the herbs that you're most likely to hear about and what they can do for your health.

Echinacea. By stimulating your immune system, echinacea increases your body's resistance to bacterial and viral invaders. "I recommend echinacea as a natural antibiotic for any age group," says Dr. Sierpina. Commission E, a government agency in Germany that reviews the safety and effectiveness of herbs, has approved the use of echinacea to help treat recurring respiratory and urinary tract infections.

Because echinacea may work by stimulating the immune response in your mouth, take the herb in a liquid form such as a tea or tincture. The typical dose of echinacea tincture would be 15 to 30 drops two to five times daily. When buying echinacea, look for standardized products that use *Echinacea angustifolia* or *Echinacea purpurea.* Start taking the herb at the first sign of cold symptoms, and keep taking it for about three weeks, Dr. Sierpina says. Do not use echinacea for more than eight weeks at a time; if you have an autoimmune condition such as lupus, tuberculosis, or multiple sclerosis; or if you are allergic to chamomile, marigold, or other plants in the daisy family.

Herbal Hops

Throughout history, men have been revered for their great ideas: Albert Einstein's theory of relativity, George De Mestral's invention of Velcro, the Dell'Aquila brothers putting herbs in beer.

Brothers Mitchell and Anthony Dell'Aquila were on the hunt for a new product for their microbrewery, the Hoboken Brewing Company in New Jersey. "Microbrews were all pretty much the same. We wanted something different that would create interest," says Mitchell Dell'Aquila. Living right outside New York City, they noticed the hot trend of city dwellers taking the herb ginseng. An idea was born, and from it sprang Mile Square Ginseng Ale.

Each bottle contains the equivalent of 200 milligrams of American ginseng, Mitchell Dell'Aquila says. That's equal to the recommended daily dosage of the herb. The beer debuted in May 1997 and has been well-received, he added.

Expect more beer to pop up with herbal ingredients. "It's an up-and-coming niche to the beer marketplace," says Doug Doretti, president of the Great American Beer Club in Lakemoor, Illinois.

Garlic. Maybe you don't have any need to keep vampires at bay, but any man would want to keep heart disease at arm's length, and garlic is the ticket for that. This all-purpose herb lowers cholesterol and keeps blood platelets from clumping together and sticking to artery walls, reducing the risk of hardening of the arteries, heart attacks, and strokes.

A study of 261 patients with high cholesterol found that 2.8 grams of garlic a day—equivalent to less than one clove—reduced cholesterol levels by an average of 12 percent.

"Garlic should be part of a man's program as he gets older. It fights high cholesterol," says Luke R. Bucci, Ph.D., vice president of research at Weider Nutritional International in Salt Lake City.

Garlic also shows promise as a natural bacteria killer. When you crush garlic cells, they turn into allicin, which acts as an antibiotic. A study of garlic's effectiveness against bacteria found that the herb showed significant activity against nearly 20 different strains of bacteria.

Out of all of the herbs, garlic is probably the easiest to find and put into your diet. Just take a walk down your produce aisle to find the herb, then toss it into a good deal of your cooking, Dr. Campanelli says. But if you want the benefits without the trademark garlic-breath smell, take garlic supplements. Use enteric-coated capsules, which pass through the stomach and dissolve in the small intestine. Follow the dosage recommendations on the label.

Ginkgo biloba. Ginkgo biloba dilates blood vessels, allowing more blood to travel through the body—especially to the penis and the brain.

In a study by German researchers, 50 men suffering from erectile dysfunction received ginkgo biloba extract for several months. All but 11 men regained the ability to have spontaneous erections.

As for the brain, the more blood that flows up there, the more oxygen and nutrients it takes along with it, which, in turn, helps you think better. "Men are always concerned with mental function. They are trying to keep that edge that declines when they age. Ginkgo can help keep the edge," says Dr. Bucci.

Ginkgo that you buy in stores should contain 24 percent flavonoid glycosides and 6 percent ginkgolides. The typical recommended dose is 60 to 240 milligrams daily. Doses above 240 milligrams may cause dermatitis, diarrhea, and vomiting. Also, the herb may increase the action of monoamine oxidase (MAO) inhibitors, such as Nardil, sometimes prescribed for depression. Don't try making your own ginkgo concoction if you have access to a ginkgo tree. The ginkgo you buy is a 50-fold concentration of the active ingredients in the leaf. And the leaf also contains highly allergic compounds.

Ginseng. Throughout history, people believed that ginseng was nothing short of a cure-all, thinking that it improved a person's resistance to stress, fought disease by building vitality, and strengthened bodily functions.

But ginseng's real claim to fame is its ability to give you an extra kick when you need it. "I like it as a mild stimulant," Dr. Sierpina says. Germany's Commission E says that the herb can invigorate during times of fatigue, sickness, and declined work performance. Use it for an added boost of energy during hectic times. But for beating constant stress and fatigue, you need take it continuously.

You'll find ginseng in all kinds of things, including chewing gum. But some products said to contain ginseng may have it in only small amounts or may contain a less effective type of the herb, Dr. Sierpina says. Make sure that the product contains American or Siberian ginseng. Dr. Sierpina doesn't recommend Korean ginseng, because he says that there is a risk of it raising blood pressure. Also, make sure that the ginseng contains between 4 and 7 percent ginsenosides, the active ingredient. The usual dose of a product containing 4 percent ginsenosides is two 100-milligram capsules daily. "In a real ginseng product, you'll notice within 15 to 20 minutes that you are more alert," Dr. Sierpina says. Ginseng is not recommended for people with high blood pressure.

St.-John's-wort. Doctors in Europe use this herb extensively to combat mild to moderate depression. The herb works several ways, but mostly it stops an enzyme that destroys "feel-good" chemicals in the brain, like serotonin and dopamine. Dr. Sierpina recommends St.-John's-wort for people who have mild to moderate depression, but who do not want to go on side effect–laden (and expensive) antidepressant medication. How does mild to moderate depression compare to severe depression? Mild to moderate depression is best characterized as a low, sad, or blue mood that persists for several weeks, months, or years. It may interfere with sleep, appetite, interest in sex, relationships, work, hobbies, and other life activities.

Only buy products that give the hypericin content, and follow the dosage directions. The daily dose is the equivalent of two to four grams of the dried herb, or one to two heaping teaspoonfuls of the herb steeped in boiling water for 10 minutes. St.-John's-wort is no quick pick-me-up; you need to take the herb anywhere from two to six weeks to notice any effect.

If you see no improvement in your mood after taking St.-John's-wort for more than six to eight weeks, you should see a doctor, Dr. Sierpina warns. And if at any time you have suicidal or dangerous thoughts, get professional help immediately. The herb should not be used if your depression is caused by substance abuse, he adds. St.-John's-wort can make a person more sensitive to the sun, so the fair-skinned should avoid excessive exposure to sunlight when taking this herb.

Saw palmetto. This extract from the dwarf palm tree berry may offer relief to the many men who have enlarged prostates, also called benign prostatic hyperplasia (BPH). As you grow older, your prostate starts to enlarge because new cells grow faster than the old cells die off. The prostate grows and slowly strangles the urethra, causing symptoms such as difficulty urinating, a weak stream, interruption during urination, and dribbling at the end. Other irritating symptoms include the sudden need to urinate and the need to urinate more frequently.

Saw palmetto is thought to control BPH

Wildcrafting in Your Kitchen

Here are some popular and easily found kitchen herbs and what they can do for your health.

Basil. Acts as a natural insect repellent that treats bad breath and headaches

Dill. Remedies colic and gas

Oregano. Fights parasitic infections and blocks the effects of carcinogens in cooked meat

Parsley. Used as a digestive aid and a mild diuretic; also combats bad breath

Rosemary. Eases digestion and stimulates appetite; also rich in disease-fighting antioxidants

Savory. Relieves gas and diarrhea and stimulates appetite

Thyme. Aids coughing and upper respiratory infections; also serves up stomach-soothing compounds that help to prevent the blood clots that cause heart attacks

---

in two ways. First, it acts as an anti-inflammatory agent, reducing the swelling of the prostate. It may also reduce the release of hormones that cause the prostate to enlarge. In Germany, saw palmetto and other plant extracts are used to treat nearly 90 percent of BPH patients.

But diagnosing BPH isn't something that you should be doing on your own. Although having BPH doesn't mean that you'll get prostate cancer, BPH symptoms can mask cancer, Dr. Sierpina says.

If you suspect you have BPH, see your doctor. Depending on your diagnosis, you can discuss the option of using saw palmetto instead of the usual BPH medications, Dr. Sierpina says. When buying saw palmetto, look for standardized products containing 85 to 95 percent fatty acids and sterols. The usual dose is 80 to 160 milligrams twice a day.

The Power of Vitamins and Minerals

Nature's Protection in Pills

Vitamin and mineral choices used to be so simple: Wilma or Fred? Barney or Dino? Now you have "maximum" formulas, "essential" nutrients, and "plus" varieties. Bottles clamor with "men's," "women's," and "seniors'" categories, never mind the "high-potency," "naturalized," and "pro-vitamins" labels found on just about every bottle in the supplements aisle of your local drugstore.

Despite the confusing jumble of letters, numbers, and some weird names, vitamins and minerals are nothing more than chemicals that your body happens to need in varying amounts. Starting in the late 1800s, scientists "discovered" and named the various nutrients. Over the past century, experts have figured out how much of each we need to ward off disease, and which vitamins and minerals are more important than others. Thus, certain vitamins have been deemed essential vitamins.

"The essential ones are the ones that, if you don't get them, you will eventually drop dead. That's how they got to be essential," says John N. Hathcock, Ph.D., director of nutrition and regulatory science for the Council for Responsible Nutrition in Washington, D.C. But we now know that vitamins and minerals go beyond bodily functions. Certain vitamins and minerals may also protect against debilitating diseases such as cancer, heart disease, and diabetes.

But if you think that vitamin and mineral supplements will offset a steady diet of junk food, think again. Nothing beats a healthy diet. "The best recommendation is to get your nutrients from food," says Priscilla Clarkson, Ph.D., professor of exercise at the University of Massachusetts in Amherst.

But combined with a healthy diet, vitamin and mineral supplements will grant you an extra edge. You'll feel good every day and feel that way for a long time, says Dr. Hathcock. Supplements will also help protect you from some chronic diseases, he adds.

Vitamins' Greatest Hits

Vitamins are nutrients that your body needs but usually can't make on its own, says Shari Lieberman, Ph.D., a certified nutrition specialist, clinical nutritionist in New York City, and author of *The Real Vitamin and Mineral Book.* Here are some of the best.

Folic acid or folate. You've heard about fats. You've heard about cholesterol. Now you have to worry about an amino acid called homocysteine and your heart health. The more homocysteine you have, the greater your risk of heart disease. But a B vitamin called folic acid or folate squashes homocysteine levels and decreases your chances of heart disease. The Daily Value of folate is 400 micrograms. Folic acid in supplement form is most efficiently used by your body. To get the same amount through food, you'd have to eat 800 micrograms of folate. That's a lot of chickpeas, broccoli, and orange juice, Dr. Hathcock says.

Vitamin A/beta-carotene. You should get 5,000 international units (the Daily Value) of vitamin A, beta-carotene, or a mixture of both daily. Beta-carotene turns into vitamin A in your body. Vitamin

A helps immune function and protects you from heart disease and cancer. The nutrient also prevents night blindness. Vitamin A is found in fish and animal foods, while beta-carotene is in carrots, sweet potatoes, spinach, and fresh parsley.

Vitamin B$_6$. You need 2 milligrams of B$_6$, the Daily Value, for proper growth and to maintain the body's structure and functions, Dr. Lieberman says. Low levels of B$_6$ have also been linked to increased heart attack risk. Vitamin B$_6$ is found in whole grains, green leafy vegetables, beans, nuts, poultry, and fish. Higher levels of B$_6$, 50 to 300 milligrams, can lower homocysteine levels, alleviate symptoms of carpal tunnel syndrome, and prevent kidney stones. B$_6$ is also therapeutic for anxiety, depression, and premenstrual syndrome, says Dr. Lieberman.

Vitamin C. Population studies have shown that people with diets high in vitamin C have lower rates of heart disease and cancer. Evidence has shown that vitamins C and E work well together. One study found that people who took both C and E supplements had 42 percent fewer deaths from all causes than did those who didn't take supplements or who only took one of the two. Dr. Lieberman recommends at least 500 milligrams a day of vitamin C. Excess vitamin C may cause diarrhea in some people.

Vitamin D. Although your body manufactures vitamin D when you're exposed to sunlight, you may not be getting 400 international units, the Daily Value, says Dr. Hathcock. And you do need it because it aids the absorption of other essential nutrients. Without vitamin D, all the calcium in the world won't do a thing for your

Too Much of a Good Thing

Despite the fact that you can buy them over-the-counter and even in cartoon-character form, vitamin and mineral supplements are potent chemicals. Use them carefully. "They can be toxic in high amounts," says Forrest H. Nielsen, Ph.D., center director of the Human Nutrition Research Center of the U.S. Department of Agriculture in Grand Forks, North Dakota.

Here's a sampling of some vitamins and minerals and how dangerous high amounts of them can be.

Selenium. People who took an average of 5,000 micrograms of selenium per day suffered from hair loss, skin lesions, tooth decay, and abnormalities of the nervous system. Even at just 200 micrograms, some people have had bad reactions to selenium.

Vitamin A. Side effects have appeared after a dose of 15,000 international units (IU), or three times the Daily Value. Side effects include headaches, drowsiness, nausea, loss of hair, dry skin, and diarrhea.

Vitamin B$_6$. Taking 2,000 to 6,000 milligrams a day over six months has caused loss of motor skills. Although some people have taken 500 milligrams a day for two years with no side effects, others have experienced toxic effects after taking only 100 milligrams.

Vitamin D. Side effects start at doses above 600 IU. Taking more than 25,000 IU daily can cause hardening of soft tissue, including the heart, lungs, and kidneys.

Zinc. People who take 100 to 300 milligrams of zinc a day have developed anemia and immune deficiency. Even doses above 20 milligrams are considered too high. Side effects include hardening of the arteries, since high zinc levels lower your high-density lipoprotein (HDL, or "good") cholesterol.

bones. Vitamin D is in fortified milk, eggs, fish, and fish oils.

Vitamin E. Among its numerous benefits, several studies have shown that this vitamin reduces heart disease risk and prevents heart attacks. Dr. Lieberman recommends a daily supplement of 400 international units for everyone. But for men who have histories of heart disease in their families or who have high cholesterol, she advises taking 800 international units a day. If you are considering taking vitamin E in amounts above 200 international units, discuss this with your doctor first. One study using low-dose vitamin E supplements showed an increased risk of hemorrhagic stroke.

Mining Your Minerals

Minerals, like vitamins, have a wide range of responsibilities, including helping the body to absorb other needed nutrients. Unfortunately, men's diets tend to come up a little short of a few key minerals. By taking either a multivitamin/mineral supplement or eating the right foods, make sure that you are getting enough of the following.

Calcium. Women usually get hit over the head with the fact that they need more calcium to fight off osteoporosis, a disease that weakens the structure of bones. But men can suffer from osteoporosis, too, says W. Marvin Davis, Ph.D., professor of pharmacology at the University of Mississippi at Oxford. Men and women over 50 need 1,200 milligrams daily, says Dr. Davis. If you don't get milk or milk products in your regular diet, calcium supplements are your best bet, he adds. You don't have to buy fancy specialty calcium supplements. Grab an inexpensive pack of antacids containing calcium carbonate as a neutralizer, Dr. Davis suggests. "Antacids like Tums are good sources of calcium," he says.

Chromium. Get 50 to 200 micrograms of the mineral through your multivitamin/mineral, says Dr. Lieberman. Chromium keeps blood sugar in check. Not having enough of the mineral may increase your chances of developing Type II (adult-onset) diabetes.

Copper. The Daily Value of copper is only two milligrams, but without it, your heart wouldn't perform up to par, Dr. Nielsen says. Copper also develops strong connective tissue and creates certain chemicals in the brain. It also aids the body in its absorption of minerals like iron. You can find copper in multivitamins, black pepper, blackstrap molasses, Brazil nuts, and cocoa.

Iron. Some research indicates that excess iron raises your chances of developing heart disease and colon cancer. Many men already eat more iron then they need each day. "Men get what they need from food for the most part. Very few have problems with iron intake," says Therese Ann Franzese, R.D., a certified dietitian/nutritionist and assistant professor of clinical nutrition at the New York Institute of Technology in Old Westbury. Look for a supplement with low or no iron. (Check your breakfast cereal; some are heavily fortified with iron, so take that into consideration when selecting a multivitamin.)

Magnesium. The Daily Value of 400 milligrams may protect you from diabetes, high blood pressure, and migraine headaches. Magnesium is in meats, poultry, dairy products, cereal, and dark green leafy vegetables.

Selenium. Stock up on this mineral—it's showing real promise as a cancer-fighter, Dr. Lieberman says. The Daily Value of selenium is 70 micrograms, and you can find the mineral in whole grains, lobster, clams, oysters, and Brazil nuts. Dr. Lieberman recommends 100 to 400 micrograms for men living in low-selenium areas—states west of the Rockies and east of the Mississippi River—and 50 to 200 micrograms elsewhere. Before you begin supplementing with more than 100 micrograms of selenium daily, discuss it with your doctor. Some multivitamins now contain selenium. If you buy additional supplements, look for selenium as selenomethionine, which is the least toxic and the most absorbable, Dr. Lieberman says.

Zinc. If you have hopes of future generations carrying on your looks, wisdom, or at least your last name, you must get enough of this mineral. Without enough zinc, your sperm count could take a nosedive. If not being able to reproduce doesn't bother you, also know that it's necessary for brain function, immunity, and wound healing. "When we look at zinc deficiency, it tends to affect males more than females," says Dr. Forrest H. Nielsen of the Human Nutrition Research Center of the U.S. Department of Agriculture. Stick to the Daily Value of 15 milligrams, which can usually be found in foods such as meat, poultry, eggs, and oysters, or take a multivitamin. "If people meet the daily requirement, they'll be all right," Dr. Nielsen says. But don't overdo it. Taking too much zinc causes anemia, damages your immune system, and interferes with your ability to absorb other minerals.

The Label Lowdown

What's in a vitamin label? Do name brands or "natural" ingredients make a difference? Not necessarily. When you're shopping for vitamins, bear the following in mind.

Natural versus synthetic. For the most part, your body can't tell the difference between the two: It absorbs synthetic and natural vitamins the same way. So go for the cheaper synthetic brands, with one exception. Your body absorbs natural vitamin E better than synthetic vitamin E, says clinical nutritionist Dr. Shari Lieberman.

Store brand versus name brand. As long as the supplement has the amounts of nutrients you need, there's no reason to buy a specific brand, says Therese Ann Franzese of the New York Institute of Technology. Many vitamin companies make both name brand and store brand. They just put different labels on them. Look on the label for the letters "USP"—United States Pharmacopeia. That indicates that the supplement should dissolve inside of you.

Multi Multiple Choice

Taking a multivitamin/mineral supplement may cover more than just the bases. A study at the Fred Hutchinson Cancer Research Center in Seattle found that daily use of a multivitamin for 10 years cut the risk of colon cancer in half. Yet another study at the same center found that multivitamin use decreased the risk of bladder cancer, as well.

Your supplement should contain the following minerals. If it has more than what we've listed here, great. But a good multi should at least have these essentials in these amounts.

- Chromium, 50 to 200 micrograms
- Copper, 2 milligrams
- Folate or folic acid, 400 micrograms
- Magnesium, 100 to 400 milligrams (People with heart or kidney problems should check with their doctors before taking supplemental magnesium. Supplemental magnesium may cause diarrhea in some people.)
- Vitamin A/beta-carotene, 5,000 international units of one, the other, or a mixture of the two
- Vitamin B_6, 2 milligrams
- Vitamin D, 400 international units
- Zinc, 15 milligrams

The Power of Supplements

A Guide to the Market

Deep in the halls of Congress one afternoon in 1994, legislators approved a document called the Dietary Supplement Health and Education Act. The act shifted to the government the onus of proving a supplement safe, whereas before, the burden lay on the shoulders of the manufacturer. Translated, it means that a product is virtually innocent until proven guilty of being a danger to your health. As long as the government hasn't found anything wrong with a supplement, it can be sold.

That doesn't necessarily mean that it works, though.

But just as you don't want to believe everything you read about supplements, you don't want to discount them either. Several have good science to back them up. Quite a few show promise, but experts don't know enough yet to recommend stocking your medicine cabinet with them.

Here, then, is a guide to the supplements that you've probably heard of and wondered about. We'll tell you which ones may actually work and which ones are just a lot of supplementary nonsense.

The Muscle-Makers

Many men would love to wake up one day built like Arnold Schwarzenegger—only without having to do all that heavy weight-lifting stuff. From this basic impulse toward sloth comes the notion—wishful

thinking would be a more accurate description—that such a body could come in a bottle of muscle- and performance-enhancing supplements.

There are two problems with that logic: First, these muscle-bound supplements don't always work; and second, you still have to bust your butt day in and day out to build a perfectly chiseled body. The following two supplements are popular among the athletic set.

Amino acids. You could shell out mega-bucks for amino acid supplements to add bulk and brawn. Or you can eat all the amino acids your body needs, by consuming chicken, beans, meat, and tuna. It tastes a lot better and bulks up your wallet. "Anyone who has a reasonable diet is going to be pretty well off for amino acids," Dr. Lemon says.

The idea behind amino acids is intriguing. Amino acids can be used for muscle fuel during prolonged exercise. Taking it a step further, you could then hypothesize that supplemental amino acid intake might enhance performance or aid in repair of exercise-induced muscle damage. But there's a problem: This is theory, not practice. "Virtually all of the amino acid ideas are theoretical. Most have never been documented," Dr. Lemon says.

One exception shows promise for athletes, but not because it adds bulk or enhances your performance. Researchers are studying the effects of the amino acid L-glutamine on the immunity of hardcore professional athletes. During heavy training, such athletes can wear down their immune responses, leaving themselves more open to infections, Dr. Lemon says. It may be that during intense training, the muscles use more L-glutamine, in effect, robbing the supply of this amino acid—an important fuel for immune function—from your immune system. Supplementing with L-glutamine could ensure that the immune system gets enough of the amino acid, thus protecting athletes from illness and infection. "There is some indication that this may help. It's not proven, but maybe we'll make that connection," Dr. Lemon says. The bottom line on L-glutamine: "Until more research is done, I would not recommend glutamine supplementation," he says.

Creatine. Denver Broncos tight end Shannon Sharpe reportedly swears by creatine. Teammate and linebacker Bill Romanowski has been quoted as saying that it can make you a better football player. Not bad from two guys who helped the American Football Conference win its first Super Bowl in years.

Several studies back up Sharpe's and Romanowski's personal experiences. Creatine has been linked to building muscle and strength, cutting down recovery time, and giving athletes more explosive power. "Some studies have shown no effect, but a number of scientific studies fall more on the positive side," says Peter W. R. Lemon, Ph.D., professor and chairman of exercise nutrition at the University of Western Ontario in London, Ontario.

A study at Pennsylvania State University in University Park gave 14 active men either 25 grams of creatine or a placebo. Those who got creatine improved their power output during jump squats and could do more repetitions during bench press sets.

Your body already produces 1½ grams of creatine daily, and you can get creatine from eating meat or fish. Either way, the creatine helps to unleash energy from muscles. The theory behind creatine supplementation is that if you have more creatine than the amount that your body makes, you

The Supplement Sideshow

Snake oil got a bum rap. It was actually considered an effective remedy for rheumatism and even toothaches and earaches. It earned its bad reputation after traveling salesmen and town frauds sold other concoctions—like lard oil—and passed them off as snake oil.

Here's an amusing list of past products touted as cure-alls, and other substances that would probably kill you before healing you. So folks, don't try these at home.

***Swamp root.* Made mostly of sugar and water colored with caramel, swamp root was touted to cure "acute and chronic diseases of the kidneys, liver, bladder, urinary organs, and . . . all uric acid troubles."**

***Hadacol.* Sold in the 1950s by Louisiana state senator Dudley J. LeBlanc, Hadacol was 12 percent alcohol, some B vitamins, iron, calcium, phosphorus, dilute hydrochloric acid, and honey. Hadacol battled "against the pain and suffering of disease." People said that it cured anemia, arthritis, asthma, diabetes, epilepsy, gallstones, heart trouble, high and low blood pressure, paralytic stroke, tuberculosis, and ulcers. It didn't.**

***The Hoxsey method.* Harry Hoxsey said that this secret method that "cured" cancer was given to him by his father—who died of cancer, but never mind. This method was made of arsenic. He would apply the arsenic paste to the cancer area, where it would eat away at the person's flesh.**

***Turpentine.* Turpentine mixed with sugar was swallowed for worms, a sore throat, or a cold.**

***Kerosene.* Kerosene was taken with a spoonful of sugar, mainly to treat colds, sore throat, and the croup. But some people claimed that it also cured pneumonia, convulsions, and diphtheria.**

could unleash more energy. You get an extra push in competition. You work out harder and faster and, therefore, build more muscle in the process. Studies have shown that you need about 20 grams of creatine—perhaps 20 times what you normally eat each day—to see an effect. "You couldn't get it in your diet unless you consumed 10 pounds of meat a day," Dr. Lemon says.

So far, no serious side effects have been reported among creatine supplement users, although anecdotal stories mention cramping, dehydration, and muscle strains and pulls from creatine use. But what we don't know about creatine is the problem, Dr. Lemon says. No studies have yet shown the long-term effect of taking the supplement daily.

But Dr. Lemon says that work in his laboratory may prove that you don't have to take creatine every day. Dr. Lemon gave 20 grams of creatine to athletes for three to five days. He then measured their performance and the amount of creatine in their muscles once a week for five weeks. Even five weeks after taking creatine, the athletes still had most of the creatine they did the week they took the supplement. Interestingly, their performance gains were also retained. "You may only need to take it intermittently as opposed to daily. It may be something that takes a much greater period of time to deplete," Dr. Lemon says. Taking only a couple grams every few weeks will also be a lot easier on cash flow, he adds.

If you decide to take creatine, be sure to take creatine monohydrate, as it is the most effective form. Stick with well-known companies to ensure quality control, recommends Dr. Lemon. The product should be at least 99 percent creatine, he says. Take it with six to eight ounces of grape juice or some other carbohydrate, he adds. The carbohydrate will stimulate a release of insulin from the pancreas, which helps creatine get into your muscles more quickly. Based on the research to date, Dr. Lemon says that a dose of about 20 grams for three to five days will maximally load the mus-

cles with creatine. Thereafter, a maintenance dose of two to three grams a day may be prudent. You can consume about one to two grams a day in your diet, however, so a supplemental maintenance dose may be unnecessary, he says.

The Heart-Helpers

Coronary heart disease is the leading cause of death, not just in American men but also in men from all Western industrialized countries. It kills about a half-million Americans a year. Up to 60 percent of those deaths are sudden. With those sobering statistics, it's no surprise that any supplement remotely linked to fighting heart disease becomes a hot item. Here are two products touted as heart-healthy supplements.

Coenzyme Q$_{10}$. Despite the futuristic-sounding name, coenzyme Q$_{10}$ (also known as co-Q$_{10}$) has been around forever. In fact, our bodies make the enzyme, and we get it from foods such as oily fish, whole grains, and organ meats like liver. Although not considered a vitamin, it acts like one because it triggers other reactions in the body. Co-Q$_{10}$ most notably aids in the conversion of food to energy.

Co-Q$_{10}$ also strengthens the heart muscle. Studies have shown that supplementing with co-Q$_{10}$ improves the health of heart disease patients and even allows some patients to stop taking heart medications. One group of researchers from Denmark reviewed eight different studies of co-Q$_{10}$ in patients who had congestive heart failure. They found that patients supplemented with the enzyme scored better—sometimes up to 76 percent better—on recovery criteria than patients who received a placebo did. "We don't have all the evidence, but when you have a heart attack, you do lose a lot of co-Q$_{10}$. It is an antioxidant, and there is something to be said for that. I don't see any reason not to take co-Q$_{10}$, as long as you're not using it as a substitute for proper health care," says Dr. John N. Hathcock of the Council for Responsible Nutrition.

Men with a history of heart problems (either in themselves or in their families) could benefit from taking co-Q_{10}, says clinical nutritionist Dr. Shari Lieberman. Anywhere from 50 to 300 milligrams a day has been used without any adverse side effects in clinical trials, says Dr. Lieberman. Capsules usually come in 10-, 30-, 50-, and 100-milligram form.

Fish oil. The fish oil buzz started with the Eskimos a few years back. Researchers realized that Greenland Inuits died less from heart disease, even though they ate as much fat as the fat-happy Americans and Danes. It turned out that the Inuits got most of their fat through fish, while we Americans got most of ours through red meat. Scientists pinpointed the difference to a certain kind of fat found in fish, called omega-3 fatty acids.

Omega-3's may work on heart disease by decreasing triglycerides, lowering high blood pressure, and keeping blood platelets from sticking together. In a study of more than 2,000 men who had just had heart attacks, part of the group was advised to eat fatty fish at least twice per week, while the rest of the group was not. After two years, there was a 29 percent decrease in death from all causes in the group asked to eat fish, compared to those who weren't.

Not everyone is convinced that you should go out and buy fish oil supplements. Eating a healthy diet that includes fish is probably just as good for you, says Lawrence Appel, M.D., associate professor of medicine and epidemiology at Johns Hopkins University School of Medicine in Baltimore.

The American Heart Association also urges that people get omega-3's right from the source. Another reason for this is that fish oil supplements can cause side effects. Some people who have taken them complain of a fishy odor and stomach upset. Other possible side effects include easy bruising, increased bleeding, and a rise in cholesterol levels.

Those people who don't enjoy the fishy taste but want the benefits of omega-3's can try other sources, such as flaxseed oil, says Gary J. Nelson, Ph.D., research chemist for the Western Human Nutrition Research Center of the U.S. Department of Agriculture in San Francisco.

Time Stoppers in a Bottle

Hormones, some believe, keep people young and free of the many health problems that come with aging. As you age, your body's production of various hormones starts to taper off; hence, the reasoning goes, you become more prone to the ravages of time. Supplement your flagging hormone levels, and you'll supposedly live longer and feel younger. That's the idea anyway. And that's why the following two hormone supplements continue to fly off the shelves.

DHEA. DHEA is the easy way of saying dehydroepiandrosterone, a hormone that is produced by your body and converted into other hormones, like testosterone. By age 60, you may have only a third or less DHEA than you did as a strapping young man. The theory is that if you replace the DHEA in your body with DHEA from a bottle, then you may put a stop to aging and all the nuisances that come with it.

As it happens, several animal studies have linked DHEA with cancer prevention, diabetes treatment, and anti-obesity, among other things. But we're talking about rats, not people. "Everything is based on animal data. Very few, if any, clinical trials have been done," says Arthur G. Schwartz, Ph.D., researcher and microbiologist at Temple University School of Medicine in Philadelphia.

Another fact that Dr. Schwartz points out is that perhaps 25 to 50 milligrams of DHEA prevents cancer in a rat, but to get that same level of DHEA in a human, you'd have to take up to 40 times that amount. "You are going to need very high doses," he says. Taking that much DHEA produces severe, possibly harmful side effects. And even at those dangerous levels, DHEA may not work in a human the way it did in a rodent. What's more, because there haven't been many long-term human trials, the experts don't know if daily supplementation of DHEA in any dosage could cause health problems down the road.

DHEA may prove to be a genuine benefit as studies of it continue. Dr. Schwartz is working on a derivative of DHEA that will hopefully have the benefits without the side effects. The DHEA-related substance will be tested for cancer prevention and treatment of rheumatoid arthritis and Type II (adult-onset) diabetes. "We'd like to show that it works at low doses, using a modified DHEA that retains the good effect and removes the bad," he says. But that's years down the road.

Melatonin. You produce melatonin in the pineal gland, a little gland found deep in the recesses of your brain. The hormone regulates your body clock, which, among other functions, tells you when it's time to go to sleep. Some believe that by taking melatonin in supplement form, you can actually control the big body clock and stop some parts of the aging process.

Despite being touted as helping with insomnia, anti-aging, and preventing cancer, melatonin's only solid track record is with jet lag. Taking melatonin supplements may help your body clock to readjust when you zoom across time zones, says Karl Doghramji, M.D., director of the Sleep Disorders Center at Thomas Jefferson University Hospital in Philadelphia. "It is somewhat impressive in some of the studies," he says. He does add that no one is sure what the right dose really is and that side effects of taking melatonin aren't well-known.

The Cartilage Connection

Arthritis is the number one cause of disability in America. More than 14 million men in the United States have arthritis, and the Arthritis Foundation estimates that by the year 2020, more than 59 million Americans could have arthritis. Several supplements have been linked to staving off joint disorders, including the following.

Glucosamine sulfate and chondroitin. These two substances, which your body already produces on its own, help build and protect the cartilage covering the ends of your bones. Using the two supplements together has shown promise as a treatment for arthritis, says Amal K. Das, M.D., an orthopedic surgeon for Hendersonville Orthopedic Associates in North Carolina. In his own study, Dr. Das gave 93 arthritis patients either a combination of the two supplements or a placebo. The supplement improved joint function and decreased the pain in those with mild to moderate arthritis. "What's really exciting is that it may actually slow down the progression of arthritis," Dr. Das says.

So far, there's nothing to suggest that taking the two can prevent arthritis and joint pain, Dr. Das says. But he recommends the combination for people with arthritis or joint pain.

Dr. Das advises taking a combination of 1,500 milligrams of glucosamine and 1,200 milligrams of chondroitin twice a day. You can buy the two separately or already combined. No side effects have been reported, but it does take at least eight weeks to take effect, he says.

Shark cartilage. This supplement made a splash a few years back as a cure for cancer. Those claims didn't pan out, at least not scientifically.

Now some experts tout shark cartilage as a treatment for arthritis, but one that's quite a bit less potent than glucosamine sulfate and chondroitin. You would have to take about two pounds of shark cartilage to get a therapeutic dose, Dr. Das says. You might as well stick with glucosamine and chondroitin if you are looking for an arthritis and joint pain treatment, he suggests.

The Power of Touch

When Healing Gets under Your Skin

Infants need more than just Mom's milk or formula to grow into strong, healthy children. They also need touch. Research has shown that babies born prematurely and even babies without medical problems benefit from one form of touch in particular—massage. They gain more weight and have lower levels of anxiety than infants who do not receive a daily massage do.

Touch ranks right up there with food and water when it comes to survival. Skin, after all, is the body's largest organ. And whether you know it or not, you already use touch to help heal. If you feel pain, you instinctively reach for where you hurt. When you need to comfort someone in either emotional or physical pain, you tend to touch him.

Thanks to the disciplines that have grown throughout the centuries, you can use something as simple as touch to give you power over stress, illness, pain, and a slew of other ailments. And unlike many other medical treatments, being healed by touch may be one of the most pleasant ways of improving your health.

Rubbing You the Right Way

The popularity of professional massage has skyrocketed in the past two decades. Between 1982 and 1992, membership in the American Massage Therapy Association increased 10-fold, to more than 15,000 people; and by 1998, membership was close to 32,000. The number of accredited training programs also jumped from 12 to 56 between 1982 and 1992 and continues to rise.

And why not? Of all the alternative therapies that have surfaced, what could be more fun and enjoyable than massage? For an hour or so, you lie undisturbed while someone gently kneads the stress and worry from your body. "Getting a massage is like taking a mental vacation. It feels good, and it is okay to feel good," says Elliot Greene, a massage therapist in Silver Spring, Maryland, and past president of the American Massage Therapy Association.

Getting a massage does more than just make you feel good. It is a powerful weapon against stress, one of the most debilitating conditions men face today. Experts estimate that anywhere from 75 to 90 percent of doctor visits are for stress-related disorders. Various studies have linked chronic stress to asthma, diabetes, gastrointestinal disorders, heart attacks, cancer, and the common cold.

A good massage allows you to let go of all the stress and worries about your job, your home, and your life. "We live in such a high-pressure, overstimulated world. A massage protects people from the ravages of this stressful world," Greene says.

Research bears this out. In one study conducted by the Touch Research Institute in Miami, massage therapists gave 15-minute massages to workers on the job twice a week for five weeks. At the end of the five-week period, the workers reported less job stress and were less depressed.

Don't assume that you'll become a useless lump of tissue after a relaxing massage. All that stroking may stroke your brain, as well. That study at the Touch Research Institute also found that after a massage, the workers completed math problems in less time, and with fewer errors, than their pre-massage selves had. "It turns out you can function better if you have reduced stress. Massage doesn't take your edge off. It may actually give you a leg up on the competition," Greene says.

Massage rubs away the aches and pains of daily living, Greene says. It relieves muscle tension and spasms and aids sore muscles after a strenuous workout. Sport massage speeds recovery time from an injury. It may even reduce injuries by loosening tight muscles and tendons that could be damaged under pressure caused by the stress of strong physical exertion.

If you are ready to throw yourself under the skilled hands of a massage therapist, the best way to find one is word of mouth, Greene says. Ask a buddy or co-worker who he likes and doesn't like. You can also contact the American Massage Therapy Association at 820 Davis Street, Suite 100, Evanston, IL 60201-4464, to request the names of qualified massage therapists in your area.

Or call a local massage school and ask for references, adds Robert A. Edwards, a licensed massage therapist and director of the Somerset School of Massage Therapy in New Jersey. Once you do find a massage expert, ask about his training, if he is a member of a professional association, and if he is licensed (if you live in a state that requires massage therapists to be licensed).

But professional massage therapists don't have a corner on the market. If you want to be convinced of the power of massage, do it to yourself first. Here are some techniques that you can employ on your own.

Just rub it. For a minor pain or soreness anywhere in the body, simply let your fingers do the walking. "Find the spot that hurts, and knead the tissue with your fingers. But if it feels very sore to the touch, either lighten up or skip that spot," Greene says. There's no special technique for this level of self-massage. It's that simple.

Make your neck nimble. This massage technique loosens tight muscles in the neck and shoulders, where a good deal of tension and stress builds up. Using both hands, grab the backs of your shoulders so that your elbows point up toward the sky, Edwards says. To a very slow count of five, move your elbows down toward the ground, while still holding your shoulders. You should feel your upper back and neck muscles lift up the farther your elbows go down, Edwards says.

Pull your skin. Place one hand on the side of your neck, as if you were holding it up. Slowly start to cup your hand and gently pull the skin away from your neck. You should feel the tension from your neck release. After doing it a few times, do it again with your head tilted downward, and then do it on the other side of your neck.

Keep the blood flowing. Sitting for a long time cuts off blood flow to your legs. Use massage to get that blood pumping again. In a seated position, cross your legs so that your right ankle rests on your left knee. Put one hand around your ankle, the other just above your knee. Move the hand that's around the ankle toward the knee with a gliding motion while applying slight pressure, and move the hand that's above the knee with the same motion toward the ankle so that your two hands meet halfway, Edwards says. Then switch legs and repeat.

Quell muscle cramps. Nothing seems to stop you dead in your tracks like a killer muscle cramp. Use massage to calm that cramp, Edwards says. Knead the area of the cramp to find the most tender spot. After finding the spot, push the skin toward the bones using both hands, Edwards says. Do this for a few seconds, then relax and repeat.

Stop sinus pain. Use your eyebrows as an outline to massage away sinus and headache pain, Edwards says. Using your index fingers, massage in a circular motion starting between your eyebrows, just above the bridge of your nose. Slowly move the massaging motion in both directions away from the nose. You should be massaging right below the eyebrows, not on the eyebrows themselves. Do this several times, Edwards suggests.

Hitting the Right Spot

Rubbing your skin is one thing. But somehow, the Western mind has a harder time accepting that sticking needles into your skin can have any kind of healing benefit. And yet, that's exactly what acupuncture does. What's more, the ancient technique has been proven effective enough to get a seal of approval from the National Institutes of Health (NIH), which conducts and supports biomedical research into the causes, cures, and prevention of diseases. The NIH says that acupuncture is especially effective in cases of post-operative dental pain, and nausea caused by surgery or chemotherapy. It also works as a complimentary treatment for other conditions, including addiction, headache, tennis elbow, muscle pain, asthma, carpal tunnel syndrome, and lower-back pain, the NIH adds.

Acupuncture and its sister technique, acupressure, are based on the Chinese idea that energy runs through a series of pathways in your body. If the energy, or *chi*, jams up or becomes too intense, you experience pain or sickness. By applying pressure to particular points, either with needles for acupuncture or with fingers for acupressure, you can fix the flow of *chi* to make a person healthy again.

Over thousands of years, practitioners of this art have learned which points on the body produce the best effects. Although no one can quite explain the scientific reason behind acupuncture and acupressure's healing powers,

Handling a Touchy Subject

It may be the only time in your life that you'll wish you were impotent.

Many men may shy away from getting a professional massage for fear they'll get an erection, says massage therapist Elliot Greene. As crazy as it may sound, it's a common fear. Some men usually get touched only during sex. So even during a nonsexual massage, their automatic reaction is to get aroused. Sometimes, it is simply a brief, involuntary reaction by the nervous system that will subside shortly.

Don't let this fear keep you from the many benefits of massage. First of all, it most likely won't even happen, he says. Second of all, if it does, and you are with a trained professional, he'll know what to do—and he won't embarrass you, he promises. "It's no big deal. A qualified massage therapist understands that it happens from time to time and can actually help somebody through it. Massage therapy basically involves relaxation, not excitation, so as a person learns to relax, the problem usually goes away," he adds. In his 25 years of professional experience, Greene says that he has learned when it is best to talk about it and when it is best to ignore it.

one theory is that the pressure triggers the release of endorphins, natural painkillers produced by your own body, says Dr. Victor S. Sierpina of the University of Texas Medical Branch.

While acupuncture works well on chronic conditions, you can't do it yourself. To find a qualified practitioner, look in the yellow pages for licensed acupuncturists, says David Nickel, a doctor of Oriental medicine; a certified acupuncturist in Santa Monica, California; and author of *Acupressure for Athletes.* You can also ask your doctor or other medical professionals for referrals, he suggests. Ask the acupuncturist about his training, how many years experience he has, and what results he has had with specific conditions.

Make sure that he uses disposable needles, Dr. Sierpina warns. You don't want somebody sticking needles—even sterilized ones—in you if they've already been in someone else.

On the other hand, acupressure is usually better suited for acute conditions. And you can do it yourself—even while sitting in traffic or talking on the phone. "If you have one hand free, you can treat yourself with acupressure," Dr. Nickel says. Here's a primer on using acupressure to help heal some typical health problems.

Grab an earful. People may think that you are doing a bad Carol Burnett impersonation, but pulling on your ear is a common acupressure technique, Dr. Nickel says. The ear contains several acupressure points that trigger healing in different parts of the body. Starting at the top of your ear, place your thumb behind your ear and your index finger on top. Lightly squeeze the thumb and the finger together. Work your way down the ear until you hit a sensitive spot. "If it's sensitive, then that's the spot. Give it a few more squeezes," Dr. Nickel says. To get the full effect, exhale about five seconds through your mouth when you squeeze the point, and inhale for five seconds through your nose while you let up.

Press down on a headache. Two pressure points on the back of your neck may put a headache to rest. The points are directly below the base of the skull, in depressions about two inches on either side of the middle of the neck. Place a thumb on each point and press firmly for 30 seconds, then release and repeat, exhaling when you apply pressure and inhaling when you let up. Or squeeze the top of your earlobe by placing your index finger where an earring would be and your thumb be-

hind the ear directly across from your index finger, Dr. Nickel says. Again, for best results, exhale through your mouth while pressing for five seconds and inhale through your nose when you let up for five seconds. For quicker results, press hard enough to feel a hot, stinging sensation at the ear point during pressure.

Before trying this treatment, Dr. Nickel suggests that you rate your headache from 1 to 10, with 10 being the worst. "Expect pain to be reduced by 50 percent or more within one to two minutes in most cases," he says. "Correctly done, this usually works faster and better than acetaminophen or aspirin and with no side effects."

Handle your head pain. Another way to short-circuit a headache is to pinch the skin about an inch into the webbing between your thumb and index finger. As you pinch it, pull on it a bit. "Keep the pressure within your comfort level," Edwards says. Sustain the pinch for 10 seconds, then take a break for a minute before repeating it on the same hand, or try it on the other hand, Edwards adds.

Push away back pain. Pressure points on either your hands or your back can help relieve lower-back pain. On the back of your hand, apply pressure about an inch above the wrist between the index and middle finger, and between the ring and pinkie finger. To use the point on your back, sit up and press your thumb into your back about a hand-width above your waistline and just next to your spine. Apply the pressure for about a minute, then switch and do the other side of your lower back, Dr. Nickel says.

Whether you're using the pressure points on your hands or your back, you want to press hard enough to feel a strong sensation—what we describe as a good hurt, Dr. Nickel says. You also want to exhale through your mouth while you're applying the pressure, and inhale through your nose while you're letting up. If your lower back doesn't feel better within minutes, or if it feels worse, then stop the treatment. And keep in mind that acupressure works better if you're not hungry or tired, Dr. Nickel adds.

A Healthy Foot Fetish

An obsession with feet may classify you as having a sexual fetish, or you could just tell people that you're into reflexology, a melding between massage and acupressure that meets at your feet. Practitioners of reflexology believe that your feet contain certain points that correspond to organs and other areas of the body. The head and sinus reflexology points are your toes. The lungs are the fleshy parts of the balls of your feet, the spine is represented by the inside edges, and so on. When you press or massage these points, you balance the body's energy and promote healing.

Reflexology can be used by itself or with massage and acupressure, Edwards says. And similar to massage, a reflexology treatment makes you feel relaxed. "For men specifically, reflexology tends to make them feel rejuvenated," Edwards says. So grab your foot and get to work.

Treat your feet. By giving yourself a foot massage, you are bound to hit the reflexology point for your problem, Edwards says. To get started, hold your foot steady with one hand, while using the other hand for massaging. Your thumb does all the work. Vary the technique by using direct pressure, circular pressure, and a gliding motion.

Touch your toes. In reflexology, remember, the tops of your toes represent your head and sinuses, Edwards says. Using your thumb, rub the very tip of your toes in a circular motion. Then work around all the toes. The rubbing should relieve sinus pain and head congestion, says Edwards.

A Healing Touch without Touching

One touch-related healing technique doesn't involve touch at all. A method called Therapeutic Touch (TT) was developed in the early 1970s by a nurse, Dolores Krieger, R.N., Ph.D., as a way for nurses to expand their healing skills, says Martha From, Ed.D., a registered nurse certified and assistant professor of community health nursing at Widener University in Chester, Pennsylvania.

The theory behind TT doesn't vary much from acupressure or other alternative therapies. TT advocates believe that we are made up of energy fields. When areas of those energy fields become congested or imbalanced, we are open to the possibility of illness or pain. Trained TT practitioners redirect or "smooth out" the energy imbalances to enhance the body's natural healing powers, Dr. From says.

A TT practitioner never actually touches a person. The patient lies or sits, fully clothed. The practitioner, usually a nurse, begins by doing a brief meditation called centering. "This is used to clear the mind of any extraneous thoughts and to allow the practitioner to be fully present to do the TT treatment," Dr. From says. Starting with the head, the nurse places her hands about three inches away from the patient and slowly sweeps down the patient's body. "The practitioner is assessing or feeling for energy imbalances through her hands," Dr. From says. The session lasts anywhere from 3 to 20 minutes, and then the patient is asked to lie down for about 10 minutes so that the full relaxation effect of the treatment can be experienced.

Several studies have shown promise for TT. One study of more than 100 patients who had undergone surgery suggests that those who received TT reduced their need for narcotic pain medications.

The Power of Sex

You Know You Need It

Is sex good for your health? Songwriters through the ages certainly seem to think so. Soul man Marvin Gaye rhapsodized about the pleasures of sexual healing, and any number of blues singers have pointed out that they don't need no doctor for their prescriptions to be filled. But these are intuitive rather than scientific reports. What do the doctors say?

"Of course sex is good for you," says James Barada, M.D., clinical assistant professor of surgery at Albany Medical College and director of the Center for Male Sexual Health, both in Albany, New York. "Men who have good, long-term sexual functioning live longer, sleep better, and enjoy generally better health and well-being."

Sex may not be healthy in quite the ways you think, however. As athletic as some especially memorable bouts of lovemaking seem, for example, the calories you expend cavorting probably won't make a dent in your love handles. "The rule of thumb is that to get a good cardiovascular workout, you need to raise your heart rate to 70 percent of its maximum capacity for at least 20 minutes," says Drogo K. Montague, M.D., a urologist at the Cleveland Clinic Foundation. "Most sexual activity isn't of sufficient duration and intensity to accomplish that goal." That's why men who are recovering from heart attacks have little to fear from resuming sexual activity, even though they may need to go easy when it comes to more strenuous physical exercise.

"Use it or lose it" is a principle that applies to the male sexual apparatus in several ways. There is some evidence that ejaculating regularly helps keep the penis, testicles, prostate, and all of the associated tubing functioning smoothly by keeping them all flushed and limber.

That's why the treatment regimen that Dr. Barada regularly prescribes for patients who have prostate or testicular infections includes having regular orgasms, whether by sex or by masturbating. "Sexual activity is the natural functioning of those organ systems, so it's a good idea to promote that," he says.

Another good reason for taking your penis out for regular spins is that cobwebs can lead to softness instead of stiffness. Erectile tissue in the male organ tends to become less pliable with age and inactivity, which makes it harder to get harder, says Irwin Goldstein, M.D., professor of urology at Boston University Medical Center. On the other hand, the more sex you have, the longer you're likely to be potent, Dr. Goldstein says.

Sex and the Whole Man

As important as it may be to keep the specific sexual cylinders firing, the deeper value of sexual healing has to do with the profound impact that lovemaking has on our entire beings—on our minds, emotions, and spirits as well as our bodies. In the deepest reaches of our brains, we are wired to be sexual beings. Fulfilling that sexual drive, especially in a meaningful relationship, creates a veritable cascade of physical, mental, emotional, and spiritual benefits.

One reason that this is true is that sex floods the system with endorphins, the body's natural pain-killing compound. That deep sense of relaxation is a boon for bodies overtaxed with stress. "Endorphins act as a natural opiate, which may be why some people really do develop sexual addictions," says Dr. Barada. "It's also why we tend to sleep so well after sex."

The psychological benefits are just as great. Sex gives you a calm I'm-on-top-of-the-world feeling that can turn a bad day into a great day in a hurry. "Sex, in general, releases tension and improves your mood," says Laurence Levine, M.D., director of male sexual health and fertility services at Rush–Presbyterian–St. Luke's Medical Center in Chicago. "That euphoric feeling can even carry on through the next day."

The flourishing business of sex therapy testifies to the fact that the opposite is also true. Men who are sexually frustrated, either because of relationship problems or physical impotence, tend to withdraw, says Steven Manley, Ph.D., a psychologist with the Male Health Institute in Irving, Texas. That leads to greater sexual frustration and anxiety, which, in turn, can develop into depression.

The Human Touch

Probably the most important reason that sex is good for you is that it represents a life-giving connection to another human being. The powerful influence that relationships have on health has been documented by numerous studies. So persuasive has the evidence become that Dean Ornish, M.D., president and director of the Preventive Medicine Research Institute in Sausalito, California, and author of *Dr. Dean Ornish's Program for Reversing Heart Disease*, who stunned the medical establishment some years back by successfully reversing heart

Sex: It Does a Heart Good

It's no picnic being one of the millions of men afflicted with some form of heart disease. Never mind that you have to give up a lot of your favorite fatty, cholesterol-laden foods. You also start to become the kind of man you swore you'd never be: cautious, tentative, slow-moving. And with good reason: Many men with heart disease have to be careful of overexerting themselves. And so they start bidding goodbye to a lot of physical activities.

Sex doesn't have to be one of them.

"Most heart patients are scared to death of, ahem, dying in the saddle," says Tommy Boone, Ph.D., an exercise physiologist at the College of Saint Scholastica in Duluth, Minnesota. "They're afraid that if they have sex, they'll have heart attacks and die on the spot." Luckily, Dr. Boone says that the link between sex and death is greatly exaggerated.

"Some doctors still rely on very old data that suggested that sex could trigger a heart attack. Those data have since been proved wrong," says Dr. Boone, who has conducted studies on sex and the physical strain it can put on the body. His results are reassuring to heart patients. "Most heart patients—unless they're in the most severe cases of heart trouble, where even walking might trigger a problem—can handle the physical effort of sex just fine." As always, if you have a heart problem, you should check with your doctor before doing any physical activity. "But if you can walk up a couple flights of stairs without hurting yourself, you can surely stand to have sex," says Dr. Boone.

disease with a program of diet and meditation, now considers love and intimacy to be the most important health factors of all. "I am not aware of any other factor in medicine—not diet, not smoking, not exercise, not stress, not genetics, not drugs, not surgery—that has a greater impact on our quality of life, incidence of illness, and premature death from all causes," he writes.

Dr. Ornish's point is not to argue that sex, per se, is good for health, but that intimacy and social connection are. Numerous studies, he says, have shown that married people live longer, with lower mortality for almost every major cause of death, than people who are single, separated, widowed, or divorced do. Married people who have cancer or heart disease live longer than single people with those problems do, he adds, while loneliness can significantly increase the chances that people will die younger from any cause.

There are, of course, lonely marriages, and they can be hazardous to health. Studies have shown that married couples who display negative or hostile behaviors have decreased immune system functions. This was true whether the couples were newlyweds or whether they had been in fractious relationships for more than 40 years.

Dr. Ornish's conclusion after reviewing this research was that the formula for good health consists of commitment, trust, vulnerability, and intimacy. "When you make a commitment to someone, you feel safer and more trusting," he writes. "You are more likely to risk being vulnerable and open to the love that longs to flow from your heart to your beloved's and back again—and the resulting intimacy can be healing."

Getting to Intimacy

Knowing that commitment, trust, vulnerability, and intimacy are good for you is one thing; making those qualities an integral part of your life is another. We will have a good deal more to say about how to accomplish this in our chapters on building a better sexual rela-

tionship (see Having Great Sex on page 97) and on fixing sexual problems (see Sexual Concerns on page 134). For now, we will leave you with three key steps toward intimacy, suggested by Dr. Manley.

Take an inventory. The first step toward developing true intimacy with another is to take an honest look at yourself, Dr. Manley says. The goal is to examine your relationship with as much honesty as you can summon, casting aside the smoke screens of self-justification and denial that cloud our thinking so much of the time. "Most of us have a tendency to avoid taking responsibility for our problems," he says. "We need to take time to look honestly at what our situation really is. Ask yourself, 'Am I dealing with my problem, or am I avoiding the issue?' Also, try to analyze what the real underlying problem is, and take a look at whether you're being honest in communicating your feelings to your partner."

Formulate a plan. Once you've taken an honest look at your relationship with your relationship, try to come up with some concrete steps toward improving it. Almost invariably in this overstressed era, Dr. Manley says, the answer may be to slow down. "If you're not enjoying your sex life as much as you want, sometimes the most important thing you need to do is rest," he says.

Ask for help. Women often joke that men will drive aimlessly around a strange city for hours rather than stop and ask for directions. Sadly, there's some truth to that stereotype, according to Dr. Manley. Asking for help tends to stick in a man's craw.

If your sexual relationship has you driving down blind alleys, Dr. Manley's advice is to stop wasting your time: Ask for help. Enlist the advice, opinions, and support of your spouse, your friends, a minister, priest, or rabbi, or, if need be, a counselor. "It takes a lot more than a hard penis to have satisfying, healthy sex," he says. "Relationships are complex, and you may need professional help to successfully address all the variables."

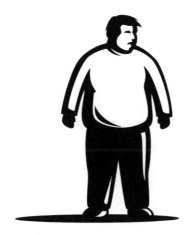

Part Three

Power Programs

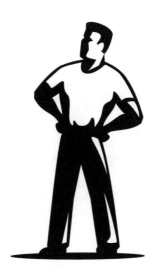

Building Muscle and Stamina

Working Out Naturally

Gym, track, basketball court, boxing ring, a weight room in the basement: Wherever bodies are being used in the pursuit of fitness is a place where holistic health is at home. Couch potatoes may blanch at the thought, but in truth, we were built to move—to lift, to swing, to run, to leap, to kick butt, if need be. Nothing could be more "natural" than working out. Indeed, what's truly unnatural is sitting at a desk inside a building all day, staring at a computer screen.

It stands to reason, then, that holistic health has a lot to offer in the way of enhancing your exercise routine, whatever your fitness goals. What follows is a program of four major steps that will help ensure that your workout is delivering the goods.

Improve the Input

You've probably heard the phrase "garbage in, garbage out." It's a maxim that fits your body as well as your software. Eat a balanced diet, and you'll get the nutrition that an active body needs. Don't eat a balanced diet, and you won't. It's that simple.

We've already devoted a the chapter, The Power of Food, to nutrition, but you'll want to take note of these few additional tips that will help keep your motors properly fu-

eled for whatever physical activity you plan to pursue.

Read carefully. In order to ensure that you get all the nutrients you need but dodge the saturated fats that can clog arteries and slow down any exercise program, a bit of homework is required. "Get used to reading food labels," says Liz Applegate, Ph.D., a lecturer in the department of nutrition at the University of California, Davis, and nutrition columnist for *Runner's World* magazine. Labels list carbohydrate, fat, and protein content in grams. An average 2,500-calorie diet, Dr. Applegate says, should contain about 380 grams of carbohydrates, 70 grams of fat, and 80 grams of protein.

Feast on fruits. Fruit is the perfect workout food. Most fruits contain lots of carbohydrate calories with no fat and very little protein, says Dr. Applegate. Fruit is also high in a form of sugar called fructose, which the body processes more slowly than glucose, the most common sugar in carbohydrate-rich foods. As a result, fruit sugars give your muscles a steady stream of carbohydrate energy over a few hours. All that, plus potassium, fiber, and vitamins.

Drink hearty. It doesn't take a genius to figure out that sweating during exercise can dehydrate your body. What many people don't know is that the best time to load up on fluids is before you get thirsty. While you're exercising, you're less likely to feel thirsty, and by the time you do, you're already in the beginning stages of dehydration, says Dr. Applegate.

To find out how much liquid you're likely to need, try weighing yourself before and after exercise. The difference is virtually all water. Each pound of water weight lost can be replaced by one pint of water, she says. So if you regularly weigh three pounds less after your average workout, try to drink three pints of water before-hand to avoid dehydration.

Scrutinize supplements. Health food stores and fitness magazines are filled with advertisements for diet supplements that will supposedly turn you into a Charles Atlas overnight. Although some supplements, such as creatine, have been associated with faster gains in strength and muscle, fitness experts agree that for basic fitness goals, you don't really need supplements if you're maintaining a healthy diet. That's especially true with vitamin supplements because a lot of foods, from breakfast cereal to white bread, are already fortified, says Nancy Clark, R.D., director of nutritional services for SportsMedicine Brookline in Brookline, Massachusetts, and author of *Nancy Clark's Sports Nutrition Guide Book.*

Asked what she thought of sports bars, Clark laughs. "I think they're 200 calories' worth of convenience," she says. "They're helpful for people who might not eat otherwise, but they're just prewrapped forms of energy. It's just putting gas in the car. Yogurt, a banana, or fig bars could do the same job."

Consider an insurance policy. In a perfect world, the vitamin companies would be out of business. But it's not a perfect world. "If you're eating a well-balanced diet, vitamins aren't necessary," says Dr. Applegate. "But that's a big assumption for a lot of people these days. They eat fast food, and they don't eat fruits and vegetables. So for people who may not be eating that well, I'd suggest a multivitamin/mineral supplement with no more than 100 percent of the Daily Value."

Gain with ginseng. One diet supple-

Meal for a Day

It's tempting to believe all the stuff you read in bodybuilding magazines, but when it comes to padding your physique with muscle, what really counts is what you eat and when you eat it.

This is a sample daily menu for building muscle.

Breakfast: Have two breakfasts. For a quick blast of protein first thing, make a quick shake in the blender, using a cup of milk, a banana, and some ice cubes. Or blend yogurt, fresh fruit, and orange juice. Then drink a large glass of water. And before you head out to work, grab something with some protein—a peanut butter sandwich, say, or graham crackers with peanut butter, and a piece of fruit.

Midmorning: If you work out at lunch, try to eat a snack two hours before you hit the gym. Aim for something with complex carbohydrates. Cereal, juice, a bagel, or toast are all good choices.

Lunch: After your lunchtime workout, your muscles are primed to store carbohydrates and ready for a little protein for muscle repairs. Get a sandwich on whole-grain bread, with turkey, chicken, roast beef, or even peanut butter again. Add a couple pieces of fruit and a few glasses of water.

Dinner: Focus on carbohydrates as your main course—pasta, potatoes, bread, and vegetables. Then, have some ice cream for dessert. You heard right: The extra carbohydrates and calories will help you maintain your weight if you are doing strenuous workouts and will keep you from pigging out late at night.

---

ment that has been working for athletes a lot longer than any energy bar on the planet is the ancient Chinese herb ginseng. Ginseng helps the body process carbohydrates and helps overworked muscles recover, says Kathi Keville, co-author of the book *Herbs for Health and Healing*. Ginseng is also said to transport oxygen to the muscles, which, in turn, helps prevent cramping, stiffness, and shortness of breath, she says.

Ginseng comes in many different forms and potencies. Varro E. Tyler, Ph.D., distinguished professor emeritus of pharmacognosy and dean emeritus of Purdue University School of Pharmacy and Pharmacal Sciences in West Lafayette, Indiana, and author of *The Honest Herbal*, recommends products containing 100 to 125 grams of standardized extract that contain somewhere between 4 and 7 percent ginsenosides. The recommended dose of a typical product containing 4 percent ginsenosides is two 100-milligram capsules daily, according to Dr. Tyler. Prolonged daily use of large amounts of ginseng may lead to insomnia, depression, headache, palpitation, hypertension, diminished sexual function, and weight loss.

We Will Rock You

Different places come with their own soundtracks. Honky tonks have country and western tunes; dentist offices have light classical; elevators have Muzak. And weight rooms often have hard rock.

The assumption seems to be that a pounding rhythm section increases the heartbeat, the production of testosterone, or both. At least one expert in the physiology of sound, though, believes that the WRR (weight room rock) format might be bad for your workout health. "You don't need heavy metal music to lift heavy metal," says Steven Halpern, Ph.D., president of Inner Peace Music in San Anselmo, California, and a composer. "When the rhythm of the music is opposite to the beating of your heart, it stresses the body. The heart has a basic rhythm we characterize as 'lub-dub, lub-dub.' It's like waltzing. The rhythm of heavy metal is usually based on a drumbeat of 'dum dum BOOM, dum dum BOOM,' with a pause after each BOOM. Compared to the natural heartbeat, this rhythm is out of sync, and it causes stress as the heart fights to maintain its rhythmic integrity," says Dr. Halpern. The sharp, percus-

Stretch Your Limits

Ask most guys to compile a list of life's 10 most boring activities, and stretching will be on it, somewhere between being stuck in a traffic jam and reading a computer manual. Yoga-style stretching is even worse because in yoga, not only are you supposed to pause before plunging into activity but also you're supposed to pause *thoughtfully*.

The good news for action junkies is that, while yoga ideally is practiced as a form of meditation, it doesn't have to be practiced that way. Even when it's done in a hurry, stretching helps prevent injury. For that reason, we asked a top yoga instructor—Larry Payne, Ph.D., director of the Samata Yoga Center in Los An-

geles—to design a stretching routine that can be adapted for guys who don't have the time (or the patience) to get in tune with the cosmos before they work out.

Dr. Payne's routine consists of four simple stretches, all of which can be completed in five minutes or less. It works for cooling down as well as warming up.

The triangle (Stretches the muscles of the upper back, chest, hips, shoulders, and neck): Take a wide stance, placing your feet 3 to 3½ feet apart, or the length of one of your legs. Your legs should be loose, with your knees unlocked and feet parallel to each other.

sive and metallic tonal quality further stresses the body, he says.

Also, the audio quality of stereo systems in many weight rooms is set up to accentuate the booming bass frequencies. The muddiness of the sound actually fatigues the body, according to research on the ear and how sound affects it, says Dr. Halpern.

"Listening to music that is improperly balanced and rhythmically out of sync with your natural heartbeat is like driving a car with your foot on the gas pedal as well as the brake pedal. You're actually working at odds with your purpose," says Dr. Halpern.

What to do? In the weight room, Dr. Halpern recommends that you request a different listening format, one that plays only light classical, nature sounds, or "contemporary instrumental music" that is "lyrical without being overly melodic."

Of course, in a weight room crowded with metal heads, insisting that the dial be switched to another station poses health risks of its own.

The quad-buster (Stretches the quadriceps and the muscles of the back, abdomen, neck, shoulders, forearms, and wrists): Sit on your heels with the tops of your feet flat on the floor. Bring both arms behind you and place your hands flat on the floor a few inches behind your buttocks with your hands and fingertips pointing forward. Keeping your hands pressed to the floor, tilt your pelvis upward, tucking your tailbone underneath you. You should feel a slight stretch in the front of your thighs.

Now, as you inhale, slowly raise your hips. Once you have raised them as high as they will comfortably go, lift your chest as high as you can. Next, slowly lower your head back, letting it hang to stretch the front of the neck. (If you feel any pain in your back or neck, skip this part of the movement.) Hold for 10 breaths, then slowly return to the starting position by doing the stretch in reverse: Lift your head into alignment with your back, and lower your chest and hips until you are once again sitting on your heels. Perform the process two times.

The lunge (Stretches the muscles of the legs and the groin, including the psoas, a deep muscle that runs from your lower back to your groin and helps in folding the body): Stand with your feet hip-width apart and take a large step forward with your left foot so that the bend of your knee forms a right angle to the floor and your thigh is parallel to the floor. (Make sure that your left knee doesn't extend past your left foot.) Your right knee will automatically lower toward the floor as you step forward. Continue to lower it until it rests on the floor. (You can place a pillow underneath if this is uncomfortable.)

Next, interlace your fingers and rest them on your left thigh. Now lift your chest, as you hold your head upward and gaze forward. To

Rest your right hand on the side of your right thigh and raise your left hand straight over your head. Keeping your left arm straight, slowly lean toward your right side as far as you can, letting your right hand slide down your leg. (This helps support the body but can also help you gauge how far you're stretching.) Hold for 10 breaths, then slowly bend back into the starting position while you breathe in for four or five seconds. Now switch your hand position and stretch to the left side. Perform twice on each side. (Tip: If you have back problems, you can bend your knees slightly. This will help take pressure off your back.)

maximize the stretch to your groin muscles, gently rotate your right thigh inward; you'll feel a stretch in your lower back. Hold for 10 breaths, rotate your right thigh back into its natural position, let go of your knee, and step back into a standing position. Repeat once more, then perform twice on the other side, stepping forward with your right foot.

The great divide (Stretches the hamstrings, Achilles tendon, and muscles of the calves, back, shoulders, and arms): Start by getting on your hands and knees with your feet and hands about hip-width apart. Without moving your feet, gently raise your buttocks into the air, straightening your legs without locking your knees. Keep your feet and hands as flat as possible on the floor. Your body should now be shaped like an upside-down V with your butt in the air. Gently lower your head as far as you can and hold for 10 breaths. Perform twice.

Working Out Mindfully

For a lot of people, any talk about there being an intrinsic connection between the mind, the body, and the spirit smacks of New Age mumbo jumbo. But many world-class athletes know that a winning attitude can pay huge dividends in their performance. If that weren't so, why bother with inspirational halftime speeches?

Here are some tips for cultivating a winning mental edge, courtesy of Eileen Udry, Ph.D., professor of sports and exercise psychology for the department of physical education at Indiana University Purdue University in Indianapolis.

Set goals. If you want to get somewhere with your training, it's important to have a plan for getting there. Dr. Udry recommends the basic "stair step" approach: Small goals lead in a logical progression to larger, longer-term goals. Writing down your goals and keeping track of your workouts can help keep you on track, Dr. Udry says. So can sharing your goals with others.

Be flexible. Don't make the mistake of being overly rigid in pursuing your workout goals. "It doesn't do you any good to stick to your program if you end up injuring yourself," Dr. Udry says. "Pay attention to what your body is telling you. Sometimes, reaching a particular goal just isn't in the cards at a given time."

Have fun. Don't be so focused on the destination that you forget the journey. If you don't enjoy working out, odds are that you won't keep working out. Different people prefer different types of workouts. Some like working out in a group situation; others like working out alone. Some like being outdoors; others prefer a gym. Some like to stick with a certain routine; others prefer novelty. "Pay attention to what works for you," Dr. Udry says.

Cool out. Stress can set you up for workout injury. That may be because stressed-out people are tense, Dr. Udry says, and therefore more predisposed to muscle strain. Or it could be that stressed-out people tend to get distracted more easily. It could be both. In any event, when the burdens of life get heavy, be extra careful when you exercise, and take steps to reduce your stress level wherever possible.

Visualize success. When you see an Olympic athlete being interviewed on TV just after he has won the gold medal, often you'll hear him say that he has been dreaming of this day since childhood. That's an example of visualizing success. Visualization is a mental exercise practiced by many, if not most, world-class athletes. But it works for casual fitness buffs, too.

Dr. Udry suggests that you visualize yourself working out as you make your way through traffic to the gym; consider it a mental warm-up period. If you're looking forward to the workout, picture yourself in the middle of it, she says. If you dread the whole routine, imagine how good you'll feel when you're finally finished.

Visualization can also be immensely helpful in recovering from injury. "Athletes can stay 'in the game' by remembering their best performances," says Dr. Udry. "That helps with timing so that when you come back to the game, you're not so much slower."

Impress Yourself

If you've ever seen a martial arts movie, you know that Asian warriors devised some pretty effective methods for hurting people and getting hurt. It's not surprising, then, that Oriental medicine has come up with some equally effective methods for avoiding injury in action and for treating injuries when they occur.

One such method that you can use yourself is acupressure, a sort of do-it-yourself form of acupuncture. You can add acupressure to your workout to warm up, cool down, and strengthen injury-prone parts of the body, says David Nickel, a doctor of Oriental medicine; a certified acupuncturist in Santa Monica, California; and author of *Acupressure for Athletes*. Here are a few basic acupressure moves to help you survive your next workout, courtesy of Dr. Nickel.

Ease into it. Acupressure is more effective if you're relaxed when you practice it, Dr. Nickel says. Find a comfortable spot, sit or lie down, take some deep breaths, and focus on relaxing your muscles. Rub your hands together to warm them up.

Make it hurt so good. Acupressure is applied with the index finger, the thumb, or both, depending on the area of the body you're working on. Press into the skin firmly enough to produce what Dr. Nickel describes as the "good" hurt. By that he doesn't mean that you should actually feel pain. "Never continue to follow a procedure that causes persistent pain," Dr. Nickel says. You should, however, feel some sensation, ranging from aching to stinging. Avoid using acupressure

Try the Healing Touch

If you injure yourself working out, acupressure can help lessen your recovery time, says certified acupuncturist Dr. David Nickel. The key is finding the right place to apply the pressure. Because acupressure (like acupuncture) works on the idea that there are channels of energy connecting various points in the body, you do not have to apply pressure to the point of injury. Instead, you want to work the corresponding point on the opposite side of your body. Thus, if you've injured your right ankle, apply acupressure to the same spot on the *left* ankle. Once you've found the spot that most closely corresponds to the injury:

- Apply very firm pressure for one minute: five seconds on, five seconds off
- Gently move the injured area as pressure is applied.
- Visualize the body part becoming stronger and more flexible as you exhale.

on bruises, scars, or any other injured part of the body.

Warm up. You can help loosen muscles during your warmup by touching an acupressure point for general muscle flexibility. The point is located on your index finger, in the crease of your first knuckle. Here is how it is done.

As you begin your stretch, use your thumb to press firmly on the point on the index finger of your left hand. Exhale through your mouth as you move into your stretch. Apply firm pressure to the point for a total of 30 seconds: 5 seconds on and 5 seconds off. As you release from your stretch, inhale through your nose and gently release the pressure on the point. Repeat on the right side. You can repeat the process once or twice. This point will help relieve and prevent muscle weakness and tenderness, too, says Dr. Nickel.

Boosting Brainpower

*Reaching into the Depths
of Your Mind*

Where you put your car keys. Your anniversary. The names of your children. That three o'clock meeting—gone. They all slip deep into the recesses of your mind, never to be found again until someone furiously reminds you that you forgot.

In this "information/technology age" you now live in, your brain has a lot to handle. But it's equipped. Your brain only weighs about three pounds, but in those three pounds lie 10,000 million nerve cells, which have several trillion potential connections with other cells. That's a wide landscape for skills, information, and memories to get lost in. But it's also a vast network containing largely untapped powers and abilities. With a little help from you, it's possible to maximize and even increase your brain's potential—naturally and easily.

Staying Bright with Bs

B vitamins, that is. Thiamin (otherwise known as B_1), vitamin B_6, and vitamin B_{12} all contribute to proper functioning of the brain. Thiamin is particularly important.

"If you dramatically reduce thiamin intake, you reduce the ability of the brain to use glucose. And if you reduce that, you have impaired mental

function," says Gary E. Gibson, Ph.D., professor of neuroscience at Cornell University Medical College at Burke Medical Research Institute in White Plains, New York. A severe thiamin deficiency not only kills the brain cells that are responsible for memory but also may cause an increase in the protein that causes Alzheimer's disease, says Dr. Gibson. The Daily Value for thiamin is 1.5 milligrams, and good food sources are rice bran, pork, beef, fresh peas, beans, and wheat germ.

Vitamin B_6 is another brain-booster. The nutrient is vital in helping to create neurotransmitters, the chemicals that allow brain cells to communicate with one another, says Michael Ebadi, Ph.D., professor of pharmacology and neurology at the University of Nebraska College of Medicine in Omaha. As a result, a lack of B_6 impairs your memory, causing trouble with your ability to register, retain, and retrieve information. The Daily Value for B_6 is two milligrams, and good food sources are bananas, avocados, chicken, beef, brewer's yeast, and eggs.

Vitamin B_{12} is essential to the production of myelin, the fatty sheath that insulates nerve fibers, keeping nerve pulses moving through your body. Without B_{12}, you're prone to memory loss, confusion, delusion, fatigue, loss of balance, decreased reflexes, and impaired touch or pain perception.

"In a severe deficiency, there is a degeneration of the myelin sheath. The stuff begins to literally erode," says John Pinto, Ph.D.,

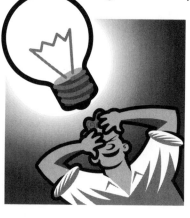

associate professor of biochemistry in medicine at Cornell University Medical College and director of the nutrition research laboratory at Memorial Sloan-Kettering Cancer Center, both in New York City. You only need six micrograms of B_{12} per day, and you can obtain that amount from eating clams, ham, lamb, cooked oysters, king crab, herring, salmon, or tuna.

The Thinking Man's Herbs

When asked about herbs that could boost brainpower, this doctor's sharp mind didn't miss a beat.

"Ginkgo and ginseng are my personal favorites. They can boost alertness and memory and improve well-being and cerebral circulation," says acupuncturist Victor S. Sierpina, M.D., assistant professor of family medicine at the University of Texas Medical Branch in Galveston.

Ginkgo biloba works by dilating blood vessels, increasing blood flow to the brain. That blood carries all of the things that help your brain function, like oxygen and nutrients. If you get more blood, you get more oxygen and nutrients, so you think better. Ginkgo also contains antioxidants, which may also increase and protect brain function.

Ginkgo has proven somewhat successful for the people who have the most problems with memory—those who have dementia. In a study of patients with Alzheimer's disease, researchers gave them either 120 milligrams of ginkgo or a placebo every day for one year. Of the ginkgo group, 37 percent had an improvement of symptoms, compared to 23 percent of the placebo group.

But you don't have to have a serious disease to benefit from ginkgo. "It's good for those of us who forgot where we put our car keys," Dr. Sierpina says. Studies in Europe have found that ginkgo improved the mental performance of healthy individuals, too.

Look for ginkgo that is standardized to 24 percent flavonoid glycosides and 6 percent ginkgolides. The recommended dose is one 40-milligram tablet three times daily, Dr. Sierpina says.

Caution: Taking too much concentrated ginkgo extract (more than 240 milligrams per day) can cause dermatitis, diarrhea, and vomiting. Also, the herb may increase the action of monoamine oxidase (MAO) inhibitors, such as Nardil, sometimes prescribed for depression.

While ginkgo may improve your memory, the herb ginseng may help you become more alert. If your brain has gone into shutdown mode—perhaps at an inopportune time like in the middle of the workday—ginseng could give you a jump start.

If you take a genuine ginseng product, you'll feel it kick in within minutes, Dr. Sierpina says. A panel of experts in Germany, called

Thinking with Your Heart

The Wizard of Oz's Tin Man wanted a heart, but the Scarecrow wanted a brain. In the very intellectual world of Western medicine, it would seem that the Scarecrow got the better end of the deal. But according to Chinese medicine, it's the Tin Man who won out.

In Chinese medicine, the brain is considered a "minor" organ, says Dr. Victor S. Sierpina of the University of Texas Medical Branch. "The brain is called the sea of marrow and does not even merit a major meridian (energy pathway) being named after it, " he says. "On the other hand, the heart is called the emperor of your body and spirit. In the Chinese view, then, the heart has a more profound influence on us than our brain does. Of course, the brain, being our thinking organ, might be trying to convince us that it is more important than our heart," he says.

We all do things at times that seem illogical and follow our heart rather than our head. "These inner readings, often called intuition, may be more rooted in heart knowledge than brain knowledge," Dr. Sierpina says.

Commission E, recommends the herb during times of fatigue and declined work performance.

Buy American or Siberian ginseng. Dr. Sierpina doesn't recommend Korean ginseng because he says that there is a risk of it raising blood pressure. Make sure that the product contains between 4 and 7 percent ginsenosides, the active ingredient. Some ginseng products have little or no active ginsenosides, so be sure to look for the percentages on the labels, Dr. Sierpina says. The usual dose of a product containing 4 percent ginsenosides is two 100-milligram capsules daily, he says.

Caution: If you do have high blood pressure, check with your doctor before taking ginseng.

Mind-Mending Melodies

Most everyone knows how just a line of an old song sends your brain right down memory lane. A good song makes you remember things you long forgot (or wish you could forget).

Music and your mental performance may also be linked in other ways. A series of studies in California showed a connection between increased memory and mental performance and Mozart's music. One study found that subjects scored better on a spatial IQ test after listening to 10 minutes of Mozart's Sonata in D Major for Two Pianos, says Don Campbell, a music therapist who lectures on the healthful benefits of music, director of the Mozart Effect Resource Center in St. Louis, and author of *The Mozart Effect: Tapping the Power of Music to Heal the Body, Strengthen the Mind, and Unlock the Creative Spirit.* Mozart may help organize the brain process, Campbell says.

But music's power over the mind isn't limited to Mozart. Depending on what you need your brain to do, here are some music selections chosen by Campbell that may light a spark.

If you are daydreaming or unfocused: Play some Mozart or Baroque music in the background for 10 to 15 minutes before you work, Campbell says. It will help you to become aware and increase your mental organization.

If you need to improvise: For those who are too analytical and need some help breaking out of the box, put on a little jazz or New Age music, Campbell recommends. This music can loosen you up and keep you from getting so uptight.

If you need stimulation, but not too much: Try some slower music by Baroque composers such as Bach, Handel, Vivaldi, and Corelli, Campbell says. The music of these composers emotes stability and order yet make for a stimulating environment.

If you need to improve concentration: Put on some slower Mozart or Haydn. The clarity and elegance of their music helps with concentration and memory, Campbell says.

Not every selection has to be "classical" to warm up your brain, says Dr. Steven Halpern of Inner Peace Music. He gives a few tips on how to choose other kinds of music to use as a mental wake-up call.

Go the instrumental route. You may think that playing your Elvis CD in the background may help you work, but then you find yourself singing softly, "Hunk-a, hunk-a burning love." When you play music with lyrics, you instinctively pay attention to the words, taking your mind off the task at hand. "The human voice and lyrics virtually force you to pay attention to them, taking such songs out of the realm of background music," Dr. Halpern says. Choose instrumental music rather than vocals as your background selections, he suggests. "Be aware, however, that if the music is very complex or 'busy,' it will also tend to call attention to itself. The net result would be distracting," he says. Therefore, he suggests choosing relaxing contemporary instrumental selections, often found in the New Age music sections of record stores.

Crank up the tunes. When Dr. Halpern feels himself going into what he calls his three o'clock slump, he turns on a different set of classics: the Temptations, Marvin Gaye, Diana Ross and the Supremes, and, of course, the Queen of Soul herself—Aretha Franklin.

"I put on Motown, and it really gets my juices flowing," he says. When your brain starts to space out, turn on whatever music gets your heart pumping. Then get up out of your seat and move your body. Dance around the room—even sing along—for a few minutes. It should get your brain back in working condition in no time.

"If you work in an office where such shenanigans would not be appropriate, listen with headphones and stretch your arms and legs, both in your chair and standing next to it. You might also visualize yourself doing the movements. Many Olympic athletes visualize in this way. If it works for them, it can work for you," Dr. Halpern adds.

Energizing Your Mind and Body

The gentle stretches and calming postures of yoga may not exactly be what you think of as a brain pick-me-up. In fact, you may think that they'd relax you enough to get you to sleep.

"But several yoga moves energize the mind as well as the body," says Mara Carrico, a yoga instructor based in San Diego, creator of *The 10-Minute Yoga Work-In* audiocassette program, and author of *Yoga Journal's Yoga Basics*.

The following yoga exercises, put together by Carrico as an energizing yoga workout, give your brain a needed boost, she says. To get the fullest impact from this energizing routine, pick a bright, well-ventilated, warm room. If you would like to have some music, choose an upbeat classical or ethnic selection. She recommends doing the workout in the morning but says that it can be done at any time during the day when you need some stimulation.

Breathing from the heart. Stand, sit, or lie on your back with your knees bent. If you're lying on the floor, place a folded towel or small pillow under your head so that your head and neck are aligned with the rest of your spine. This makes the position more comfortable. Place one hand on your stomach, the other hand on your chest. Breathe into your heart as you inhale, expanding your chest. As you exhale, let your chest relax and your stomach flatten. Continue for 5 to 10 breaths. For a more energizing effect, make your inhalations longer than your exhalations.

Half-tortoise. Kneel on the floor and bend forward so that your torso rests on your thighs, your forehead is on the floor, and your arms reach forward. Lengthen your torso as you reach forward. Keep your elbows straight and your palms flat on the floor with your fingers spread. Hold the pose for several breaths.

Cobra. Lie on your stomach with your arms bent so that your hands are beneath your shoulders. Keep your legs hip-width apart. Inhale and slowly lift your upper body by straightening your arms. Your elbows should stay slightly bent, but don't hunch your shoulders. Keep them down from your earlobes. Your buttocks are tight, with your hips, legs, and feet on the floor. Look forward or up. Hold the pose for 10 to 20 seconds. As you slowly lower yourself down, exhale. Repeat two or three times.

Downward facing dog. Get down on all fours with your hands underneath your shoulders and your knees underneath your hips. Flex your feet and tuck your toes forward. Then lift your knees until you form an inverted V. Lift up on the balls of your feet and straighten your legs, making your buttocks the high point. Keep your elbows and knees straight but not locked, and let your head and shoulders relax. Then, finally, press your heels toward the floor. Hold the pose for several inhalations, then return down onto the floor on all fours. Repeat two or three times.

Breath of fire. Kneel on the floor with your feet tucked underneath your buttocks and your hands resting on your thighs. You can also sit in a chair with your feet flat on the floor. Take a deep breath in. Tighten your abdominal muscles sharply and blow the breath out by rounding your lips—as if you were blowing out candles on a cake. Each exhalation is quick, lasting only about a second. Blow out 20 to 40 times. Your inhalations will take care of themselves while you are doing this. Afterward, rest and breathe slowly for a few breaths. Then perform the exercise again.

Taking a Chill

In this fast-paced, deadline-oriented world, a lot of people equate stress with better performance. It seems that if you aren't stressed out enough, you probably aren't doing such a hot job.

Wrong, says Elliot Greene, a massage therapist in Silver Spring, Maryland, and past president of the American Massage Therapy Association. When you relax, your mind enters a state in which it thinks more clearly and works more productively. Under stress, the brain doesn't function as well. Reducing stress gives you a mental edge over others. Here are some quick and enjoyable ways to take some stress off and boost your brain at the same time.

Take a whiff. "Basically, any essential oil that you smell will give you a mental boost," says Michael Scholes, president and founder of the Michael Scholes School of Aromatic Studies in Los Angeles. But a few essential oils pack a special brain wake-up call, he adds. Try peppermint, basil, and rosemary when you need to improve your brainpower and alertness. You can buy products such as candles or a diffuser to emit the scents around your office.

Point in the right direction. With the tip of your finger, you can give your brain a jolt, says certified acupuncturist Dr. David Nickel. The brain point in acupressure lies right at the upper tip of your earlobe, about where the ear canal starts. Pressing the brain point maximizes both your physical and mental performance, Dr. Nickel says. Hold the upper tip of your earlobe between your thumb and forefinger, and press for five seconds, then let up for five seconds. Repeat this for about a minute, he advises.

"For better results, exhale through the mouth while pressing and inhale through your nose as you let up. Also, pinch the ear hard enough to feel a 'good hurt' (hot stinging sensation). This 'good hurt' lets you know that your brain has been adequately stimulated from the nerves in your ear to turn on brain messages (neurotransmitters) and hormones for optimal performance," Dr. Nickel adds.

Dr. Nickel also notes that you should expect your best performance several minutes after pressing the brain point. "In training master swimmers, 60 percent of the time they did their personal best only minutes after using the brain point," he says. "You should expect an improved sense of well-being and control in less than one minute when correctly using the brain points."

Try another acupressure exercise three times per day to boost your brain production: Place your fingertips on your temples. Breathe deeply as you apply firm pressure and rotate your fingers slowly for one minute, says Michael Reed Gach, Ph.D., founder of the Acupressure Institute in Berkeley, California, and author of *Acupressure's Potent Points*. "This will help increase your brainpower and boost your memory," Dr. Gach says.

Massage the mind. A massage may take the stress edge off, but it may also give you an extra edge when it comes to using your brain. A study at the Touch Research Institute in Miami found that after massages, workers completed math problems in less time and with fewer errors. Massage helps you enter a more relaxed state, says Greene. If your personal massage therapist is booked, try some self-massage.

Having Great Sex

Learning the Language of Love

If learning how to make love is an educational process, then tantric sex is the Ph.D. program. Tantra is based on ancient Hindu spiritual teachings in which sexual love is considered a form of spiritual sacrament. "It's a system that can elevate a couple's sexual relationship to the level of art," says Charles Muir, a long-time teacher of Tantra, director of the Source School of Tantra Yoga in Paia, Hawaii, and co-author of *Tantra: The Art of Conscious Loving.*

Tantra combines classic Eastern spiritual principles with very practical suggestions for heightening the sexual experience. Sex is seen as a vehicle for achieving a higher state of consciousness in which the poles between male and female ultimately dissolve, resulting in unity and bliss. Key to reaching that state of bliss is maintaining a state of balance and sharing energy. "It's like going up a scale. You think, 'This is what sex is.' Then suddenly your pleasure goes up to a higher level and you realize, 'Whoa. This is better than I imagined,'" says Muir.

That's a moment we probably all hope for in our sex lives, and tantric sex is just one alternative method that you can use to seek that moment out. Many of the other disciplines and practices we talk about in this book—massage, herbal remedies, and aromatherapy among them—also can help you ensure that your next sex is your best sex. We'll look at each of the different methods in turn.

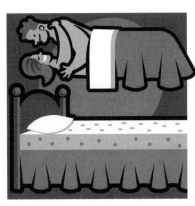

Talking Tantra

The sticky part of tantric sex for a lot of men is that ejaculation is postponed as long as possible. Some men can have sex for hours without having an orgasm and may not ejaculate at all during a given session of lovemaking. The reason for this is that ejaculating supposedly depletes the sacred sexual energy. "The man of Tantra discovers that he's most empowered just before ejaculation and orgasm. The trick is to learn to ride the wave rather than letting it crest," says Muir.

Muir is aware that this kind of delayed gratification doesn't fit very comfortably with the go-for-it mentality of Western man, as much as Western women may like it. "All I can say to the doubters is, 'Gather data,'" he says, laughing. "If you give a man an experience or two, he soon sees for himself how powerful Tantra is."

If you're game to try, here are three basic techniques of tantric sex that Muir recommends.

Give her the gaze. More than anything, tantric sex is about achieving true intimacy between lovers. If the two sexes are to achieve a higher state of unity, male-female barriers must dissolve.

A key step toward that goal, Muir says, is simply to lovingly gaze deep into one another's eyes while making love. "Closing eyes shuts out the lover and creates darkness during a potentially enlightening experience," he says.

Exercise the love muscle. The next time you're in the men's room, try shutting off your urine in midstream. The muscle you contract to do that is the pubococcygeal muscle, or PC for short. Squeezing and relaxing that same muscle during sex can help you avoid ejaculating, says Jack McAninch, M.D., chief of urology at San Francisco General Hospital.

The PC muscle can be strengthened with exercise. Practice clenching it tightly for 3 seconds at a time, giving the muscle one extra squeeze before letting go. Relax for 3 seconds and repeat the exercise. As you get stronger, gradually increase the length of clenching time to 10 seconds before the final squeeze and release, making sure to relax the muscle completely between contractions.

Breathe together. As with other forms of meditation, controlled breathing is a key part of tantric sex. The next time you're making love, try slowing down as you approach orgasm, rather than speeding up, by holding your breathing and your movement. Move and breathe in and hold for a few seconds, then move and breathe out. As the moment of release nears, clench your PC muscles, lie still in your lover's arms, look into each other's eyes, and try to match your breathing with hers. Expect to ascend.

Other Paths to Ecstasy

In addition to tantric sex, there are numerous other alternative options to excite and entice one another and enhance and enrich your lovemaking. Some of these methods may sound familiar to you. Indeed, you may have been using them all along—in which case, you won't have any trouble expanding your imagination a little bit to include these variations on a sexual theme.

Sniff out romance. To enhance your lovemaking, try using the essential oils that aromatherapists say most effectively stimulate sexual response.

Tops on the list for turning men on are sandalwood and jasmine—especially jasmine. "If the rose is the queen of fragrance, then jasmine is the king," says Victoria Edwards, an aromatherapist in Fair Oaks, California. Her choices for the scents most likely to send a woman over the edge are vanilla and cinnamon. Other scents that have aphrodisiac qualities, she says, are black pepper, ylang-

ylang, cardamom, clary, patchouli, neroli, clove, and rose.

Any of these scents can be used alone or mixed together into a love potion that best suits you and your partner. Whether diffused through the room, in a bath, or in some massage oil, they'll definitely help transport both of you to a more sensual place. All oils should be diluted in water or a carrier oil (like a massage or vegetable oil) before being used.

Caution: Never use cinnamon or clove oils in the bath. Used in large amounts, they can actually be toxic.

Rub it in. If you're serious about setting the scene for sex, take the next step by taking time for a sensual massage.

Massage therapists stress that while massage can be used as a part of sexual foreplay, the two are not synonymous. "The goal of massage is to relax, not stimulate or excite," says massage therapist Elliot Greene. "Nonprofessional massage in a sexual context prepares you for foreplay by causing you to be receptive, physically. It helps clear your mind of the stresses of the day and allows you to focus on what's happening with your body."

Practice your strokes. There are three basic types of strokes used in massage, says Greene. Try these.

- Long, smooth, gliding movements using a flat hand (called effleurage) are ideal to start with because they gently warm up your partner. The amount of pressure applied can vary.
- Kneading strokes (called petrissage) are for working specific muscles and joints. Keep your palm flat on the body and "knead" your partner's skin like bread dough, gently, with your fingers and thumbs. If you come across an especially tight knot of muscle, press your thumb into it gently and rotate to loosen the knot. These are called thumb presses.
- Percussion strokes (called pepotement) use the sides of the hand to tap the skin,

fast or slow, with hard beats or soft. These work best on your partner's fleshier regions, such as the thighs or buttocks.

Using these strokes as your basic building blocks, you're now ready to assemble the perfect massage. A good structural model to keep in mind is the pyramid: Start with broad, easy strokes, gradually tighten your focus down to specific muscles, then work your way out again. And don't forget the massage oil.

Touch her from head to toe. The specific itinerary of a massage is a matter of personal taste, and it can always be varied. Here's one route recommended by Greene. (For the face, feet, legs, hands, and arms, your partner should be lying on her back. After massaging these areas, have your partner turn over onto her stomach and massage the backs of the legs, neck, shoulders, and back.)

- The face: Starting a massage with your partner's face will establish an immediate sense of intimacy and tenderness. Use some gentle thumb presses beginning at the bridge of the nose and moving out along the eyebrows to the temples.
- The feet: This is finger-work territory, and it's probably as sensitive an area as any on our bodies, along with the hands and the face.
- Hands and arms: Kneading works well on the arms. For the hands, use your fingers, rubbing thoroughly along each of your partner's fingers and palms.
- The legs: Kneel beside your partner to work on the legs, which are well-suited to kneading strokes. Work up the thighs to the buttocks and down again.
- The shoulders and neck: Along with the back, the neck and shoulders are the

Go, Goddess, Go

It's not necessary to buy into the philosophical underpinnings of tantric sex to benefit from its practical applications. Nonetheless, perhaps you should be aware that tantric teachers think that the world is coming to the end of the Age of Darkness and that we stand on the cusp of the Age of Truth.

The main event of this new era will be the awakening of the goddess Shakti, who has been sleeping for the past 2,000 years, give or take a century or so. There's evidence of this awakening in the women's movement, according to Charles Muir of the Source School of Tantra Yoga. The goddess is shaking the sleep from her eyes, Muir says, and soon her radiant energy will "illuminate all humankind."

How should men react to all this? Go with the flow, says Muir. "This isn't about taking energy away from the man," he says. "It's about the sexual energy of both the male and female being multiplied. If I can assist my woman in awakening, more of her awesome sexual Shakti—sexual energy—shines on me as well as on her."

main event in any massage. After some warm-up strokes, knead the shoulders, starting from the outside and working in toward the neck. Rub with your thumbs on either side of the neck, then work your way back out toward the shoulders. Repeat several times.
- The back: Use long smooth strokes all the way from the shoulders down over the buttocks, as if you were finger-painting your partner's back. Then you can start concentrating on specific points of tension with kneading strokes and finger presses.

Losing Weight

The Battle of Your Bulge

If you count yourself among those who could stand to lose a few pounds, you are not alone. More than 78 million Americans weigh more than 20 percent over their ideal weight, which is the general definition of obesity. Americans spend $30 billion a year on weight-loss programs and diet products. The popularity of weight-loss drugs exploded, only to be brought back down to Earth (for awhile) after tests revealed that they may damage the heart.

Meanwhile, there is a natural way to lose weight, without pills and shakes. From your food choices to acupressure to your sense of smell, you can design your very own weight-loss program that will shed the pounds without requiring you to take medication or compromise your lifestyle.

Feeding Your Needs

If you are looking for a "natural" aid for weight loss, it doesn't get any more natural than eating a plant-based diet. If you are a normal American, you can find what you need for weight loss in any supermarket—provided that you steer clear of the junk-food aisles and focus more on aisles where you'll find the good stuff, like produce and grains, says G. Kenneth Goodrick, Ph.D., assistant professor of medicine at the Baylor College of Medicine in Houston.

When it comes to your food choices, don't take the deprivation angle. That will just make you lust for food even more. "Instead, focus on what

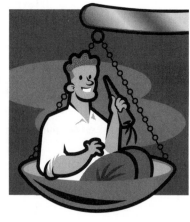

you can eat for better health. The wonderful new food choices and creative combinations of grains and vegetables that abound today are unparalleled in history," says Robert Cullen, R.D., Ph.D., assistant professor of food and nutrition and nutrition, and dietetics program director at Illinois State University in Normal. Here are some examples.

Reach for fiber. One word: apples. Okay, another word: carrots. When you need to snack or have a dessert, eat one of those, or any high-fiber fruit or vegetable. Fiber fills you up, making you less likely to pig out on less healthy food fare. A study at the Brooke Army Medical Center in San Antonio, Texas, found that eating pectin, a soluble fiber found in the skins of fruits and vegetables, made people feel full longer. Push for 25 grams of fiber a day, says Dr. Victor S. Sierpina of the University of Texas Medical Branch. "Fiber is always a good choice for a snack," he says.

In addition to their filling properties, high-fiber foods tend to be naturally low in fat and calories. "If you are not eating any fiber, it means that you are probably eating fat, because foods such as fish, chicken, and red meat, which have no fiber, do contain hidden fat," says Neal Barnard, M.D., president of the Physicians Committee for Responsible Medicine in Washington, D.C., and author of *Eat Right, Live Longer*.

Go low. If you eat foods high in fat, you get fat. It's that simple. To maintain a healthy weight, the American Heart Association recommends limiting your fat to 30 percent of your total daily calories. Eating a diet high in fiber and loaded with fruits and vegetables helps limit your fat intake, Dr. Sierpina says. Watch your use of oils and butter, and look at the fat grams on food labels. Switch to lower-fat dairy products such as skim milk and low-fat yogurt.

Also, you may have to

control your carnivorous instincts. "Don't eat too much meat. If you eat meat, make sure that it is lean meat," Dr. Goodrick says. Stick to leaner cuts such as tip round, bottom round, and top sirloin.

And limit yourself to three ounces a day—about the size of a deck of cards or the palm of your hand.

Stick with the plants. It bears repeating, so we will: By eating a diet full of fruits and vegetables, you eat more fiber. It's good for weight loss because it makes you feel full. And if you are eating lots of fruits and vegetables, you're probably eating less fat. To get more vegetables in your diet, make them the center point of each meal. Fill at least half your plate with vegetables, says Dr. Sierpina.

A Test of Wills

Losing weight comes down to a war of wills—yours and yours. You want to shed some pounds, but you also want that pepperoni pizza and six-pack. You promise to make your snacks healthy, but your mind tells you to go ahead and eat that bag of chips.

You need your mind to safeguard against itself in your battle to take off and keep off the pounds. Here are some ideas to prepare for the mental challenges that you may face during your journey to a sleeker you.

Relax, don't eat it. Stress can make us do things that we really don't want to do—like eat an entire box of chocolate-covered donuts in 10.6 seconds flat. Under any other circumstances, you wouldn't do such a thing. But stress creates a whacked-out connection between your mind and your

No Magic Pill

It's tantamount to the search for the Holy Grail and the hunt for the Loch Ness monster: the quest for a pill that makes you lose weight.

"As far as I know, there is no scientific research validating any supplement assisting in weight loss," says Dr. G. Kenneth Goodrick of Baylor College of Medicine.

Supplements such as pyruvate, chromium picolinate, phenylalanine, and chitosan claim to do everything from absorbing fat before your body can to suppressing your appetite. Although some may have the potential to work, no one has proven them to work, and no one is sure of the health risks of these substances, Dr. Goodrick says. "I wouldn't recommend them," he says.

One herb supplement touted as a weight-loss aid has proved dangerous. The herb *ma huang*, also known as ephedra, opens up air passages and is often used to treat bronchial conditions. But it also acts as an appetite suppressant and speeds up your metabolism, making it a popular diet supplement. The Food and Drug Administration has received more than 800 reports of bad reactions to the active ingredient in ephedra—ephedrine—including strokes, high blood pressure, heart palpitations, and heart attacks. It was also linked to 36 deaths. "Anything that jazzes up your metabolism is not going to be a good idea," Dr. Goodrick says.

Basically, no pill—even if scientifically proven to help aid weight loss—will ever help you if you aren't following the tenets of weight loss: exercise in combination with a low-fat, high fiber, plant-based diet. "Exercise should be the foundation. And you should eat like primitive man—lots of fiber, not too much meat, and lots of fruits and vegetables," Dr. Goodrick says.

stomach, with the former ordering the latter to consume everything in sight.

When you feel the need to feast under stress, take a break for a quick breathing exercise, says Larry J. Feldman, Ph.D., director of the Pain and Stress Rehabilitation Center in New Castle, Delaware, and author of *Feeling Good Again*, a self-help book for dealing with stress. Inhale, and when your lungs feel naturally full, take in even more air. Exhale soon after you completely fill your lungs. After you exhale, push out more air to a count of 10 until you have completely emptied your lungs as much as possible. Then start the process again by inhaling. Do this exercise five times, then rest two minutes, and repeat. This breathing exercise will help you relax, release tension, and increase concentration and willpower, Dr. Feldman says. "Weight loss is all about improving brain function to enhance willpower. Your brain function is improved, and thus your willpower increased, when your stress level is reduced."

Get a little help from your friends. Don't try to lose weight alone. Find a friend to come along for the ride and you'll increase your odds of victory. "All the studies show that people who have the best success are those who have support," Dr. Goodrick says. Women do this better than men, he adds, so we could all take a lesson from them. While women freely talk with other women about their weight-loss goals and problems, men tend to keep it inside or make it a competition. Enlist someone—a coworker, your partner, a family member—to go on a weight-loss program with you. And rely on that person as a partner, not an opponent.

Set your eyes on the prizes. Although losing weight may be your primary goal, it shouldn't be your only goal. Just focusing on how many pounds you lose and how fast you lose them may doom you to failure. "Many people become weight-obsessed and become depressed if they don't lose enough weight. If you don't lose weight soon enough or you have some trouble, you could become discouraged and stop," says Nicholas Hall,

Ph.D., director of the Institute for Health and Human Performance in Tampa, Florida. Set other health-related goals that come along with becoming fit and losing pounds. As you meet these goals, you'll be rewarded and keep on your quest to lose weight. Here are some of Dr. Hall's goal suggestions.

- Lower cholesterol levels
- Lower blood pressure
- Reduced body fat percentage
- Fewer sick days taken
- Increased distance and time you can walk or run

A Few Pointers

You use your fingers to point at the food you want, and you use them to get that food into your mouth. Now you can use them to stop your hunger pangs. The ancient art of acupressure contains several points to curb hunger and to control stress, which can trigger an eating episode. Get ready to let your fingers do some walking.

Close your ears. Place your finger on the harder part of your ear near your cheekbones. Hold that part of your ear between your thumb and forefinger and press. This is the hunger acupressure point on the ear, says certified acupuncturist Dr. David Nickel. Pressing this point should help control compulsive eating, which will help you lose weight, he adds. Hold the point for five seconds, then let go for five. Continue these five-second intervals for about a minute. "By pressing the hunger point strongly, you will stimulate the brain to release morphinelike chemicals that are able to reduce stress, induce a feeling of well-being, and reduce the compulsion to eat sweets and nutrient-depleted food," Dr. Nickel adds.

Dr. Nickel notes several cautions about using the hunger point: It is best not to use the hunger point or to only press very lightly if you feel full or very hungry, or if you are administering acupressure to a young child or infant. "Avoid pressing on a skin surface that has a scar, infection, or any previous soreness," Dr. Nickel adds. He also recommends stopping treatment if no relief is observed.

Press the "appetite balancing point." You may reach for food when you are out of balance, which can be caused by stress or any number of things. A point right above your upper lip restores balance and curbs your appetite. "It has a calming and centering effect," says Dr. Michael Reed Gach of the Acupressure Institute. Place your fingertip in the center of your upper lip, about two-thirds of the way up between your lip and nose. Press firmly, pushing into you gums, and breathe deeply. Hold the point for about two minutes. "The more often you press this point, the better and faster it will work," Dr. Gach says.

Reach for the pit of your stomach. Some people confuse pent-up stress with hunger, Dr. Gach says. "Many of us hold tension and stress in our stomachs. When they accumulate there, there's a feeling similar to hunger," he says. The following acupressure point in your stomach releases that stress and tension. Midway between the bottom of your breastbone and belly button lies a point for releasing tension in the pit of your stomach. With your fingers curved inward slightly, place your fingertips at this midway point. Slowly push into the point as you lean forward. Breathe deeply as you apply pressure to this point. Don't hold for more than two minutes, and don't push into this point after you eat, Dr. Gach warns. "Go into this point very gradually," he says. Use it for stress prevention and relief.

Yoga and Your Weight Loss

The calm flowing postures of yoga may not equate with the sweaty pounding aerobics normally associated with losing weight. But yoga can be an effective tool if you want to drop a few pounds. "Indirectly, yoga can certainly be a weight-loss exercise," says Aladar Kogler, Ph.D., director of the Columbia University Sports Psychology Laboratory in New York City, five-time Olympic fencing coach, and author of *Yoga for Every Athlete*.

Yoga can help you to lose weight in several ways, Dr. Kogler says.

- It builds energy. The postures and practice of yoga increase the amount of energy you have, Dr. Kogler says, making you more vitalized to get exercise and help you lose weight.

- It helps you develop self-discipline. "The methods used in yoga are very useful for self-regulation. The methods of concentration, meditation, and breathing all teach self-control," Dr. Kogler says.

- It fosters a healthier lifestyle. Many people who take up yoga find themselves eating healthier and exercising more, Dr. Kogler says. Yoga brings about an awareness of your body and makes you more in tune to keeping it healthy.

- It activates the endocrine system of your body. Yoga stimulates and regulates the production of hormones in your body, thereby helping to regulate your metabolism, which is a factor in controlling your appetite. "In this sense, yoga would be a help for controlling weight loss," Dr. Kogler says.

Dr. Kogler advises that those new to yoga start out with a beginners' yoga class, where they will learn the basics. He says that you can get a list of certified yoga teachers in your area by writing to the Himalayan International Institute of Yoga Science and Philosophy at R. R. #1, Box 400, Honesdale, PA 18431-9706.

Reducing Stress

How to Calm Down

Reducing the stress in your life is a lot easier than you think. In fact, we've narrowed it down to four simple steps.

Step One: Get rich.

Step Two: Quit your job.

Step Three: Move to the Caribbean.

Step Four: Hire Jimmy Buffet to perform for you every night.

Since most of us can't get as far as Step One, we have to devise other ways to take some of the stress out of our lives. Although some stress helps you handle whatever dilemma is at hand, constant or uncontrolled stress hampers everything in your life. Stress affects everything from DNA repair to interpersonal relationships, says Dr. Nicholas Hall of the Institute for Health and Human Performance. "If one doesn't control stress, everything else becomes more difficult."

Stretching Away Stress

"The relaxation poses of yoga slow down the body's nervous system and allow you to shift gears. A few poses during a stressful period could be all you need to center yourself and reduce the hold stress has on you," says yoga instructor Mara Carrico.

Carrico devised a quick and simple yoga routine to help you relax and unleash your stress. To get the most out of a relaxing yoga workout, find a quiet, calm place. She recommends practicing these exercises in the afternoon or evening after a busy day, although you could do them at any time. "These

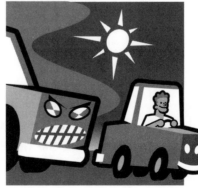

poses bring about relaxation and flexibility," she says. "Take it at a slow pace, resting for several moments between each exercise."

Four of the following five poses are while you lie on your back. For greater comfort and neck alignment, place a small pillow or folded towel under your head.

Breathing from the belly. Lie on your back with your knees bent, your feet hip-width apart and flat on the floor, and your hands on your stomach. Breathe into your abdomen—expand your belly as you inhale and contract the belly as you exhale. Take 5 to 10 breaths.

Two-legged platform. Lie on your back with your arms at your sides, your knees bent, and your feet flat on the floor. Slowly roll your spine up as you exhale, starting with the tailbone. Your buttocks and lower back will come off the floor, forming a slanted line or platform from your knees down to your shoulders. Your neck, shoulders, upper back, and feet should stay on the floor. Hold your hips and buttocks up as you inhale. Then as you slowly lower yourself back down, exhale. Repeat this exercise three to five times.

Knee to chest. Lie on your back with your arms at your sides. Bring your right knee to your chest and clasp your hands beneath your knee. Relax your right foot. Your left leg is straight on the floor with that foot flexed. Center your head and relax your shoulders. Hold your knee to your chest for 20 to 60 seconds, then switch to the other side. If you have time, do another set.

Supine leg stretch. Lie on your back with your legs straight and arms at your sides. Bring your right knee to your chest and place a strap or a belt around the ball of your foot, keeping one end of the strap in each hand. Exhale as you slowly straighten your leg toward the ceiling. Keep holding the strap and gently pull your leg toward your body. Also keep your left leg straight on the floor and flex your left foot. Hold the stretch for 30 to 60 seconds. Switch to the other side and repeat the exercise. If you have enough time, do another set.

Yoga mudra. Sit on the floor in a cross-legged pose or in a chair with your feet flat on the floor. Grab either wrist behind your back, sit up, and inhale. As you lean forward about 30 degrees, exhale. Suspend the breath, holding it out, not breathing, as you stay in this position for three to five seconds. Inhale as you return to your starting position. Exhale again, staying upright. Try three to five sets of this exercise. To make this exercise more calming, exhale for longer than you inhale. For example, if you breathe in for four to five counts, breathe out for six to eight counts, Carrico recommends.

Soothing Songs and Sounds

Music can calm the savage breast, especially if the savage breast belongs to you, when you find your stress levels rising during a high-stakes meeting or while crawling through rush hour traffic. "The right kind of music can provide a mini-vacation, an oasis of serenity no matter where we are," says Dr. Steven Halpern of Inner Peace Music.

You don't have to lull yourself into a half-comatose state by listening to boring, bland elevator music. Use many different styles of music many different ways to get your stress levels down. Here's how.

Feed your head. For those of you lucky enough to have your own office and a door, it's not that hard to play music during the workday. If you're in a cubicle, invest in a pair of

It's a Stress-Free World After All

The new mantra for stressed-out people could become "I'm going to Disney World."

The company that gave us a happy talking mouse and endless strains of "It's a Small World After All" has created a town with its very own stress-recovery program and stress consultant.

Celebration, Florida, is a planned community built by Disney near its Disney World complex in Orlando. About 1,500 residents live there now, and there is a total of 8,000 residences. Located near the center of town is Celebration Health—a state-of-the-art health, wellness, and fitness center/hospital. "Celebration City is basically an entire community designed to foster healthy mental and physical living," says the Institute for Health and Human Performance's Dr. Nicholas Hall, a consultant for Celebration.

A cornerstone of the Celebration Health Center is the eight-week stress-recovery program co-designed by Dr. Hall and Dick Tibbits, Ph.D. Residents and anyone else who is interested (program participants include several corporations) take part in nutritional consulting, cognitive therapy, exercise programs designed specifically for stress, and a host of other programs, including one that deals with spirituality and stress. "We work with people to identify personal goals and professional goals and how they can meet those goals," Dr. Hall says.

At its first stress-recovery program, Hall says that 37 showed up, even though originally the class was going to be limited to 20. "It was extremely well-received. People have been lining up," he says. No sign of Mickey Mouse or Donald Duck signing up yet.

headphones, Dr. Halpern says. Either way, plug in your favorite relaxing tunes when you feel the stress bearing down on you. Even if you can only manage a few minutes of private musical bliss, it will at least knock you down a few stress levels, he says.

Bang on the drum all day. Todd Rundgren said it best when he wrote the song "Bang on the Drum All Day." When you feel the pressure, take a pencil or pen and go to town on your desk, computer, or whatever gives you a good beat. "Make your own music," Dr. Halpern says. The drumming gets a musical flow going, and it also allows you to get out your frustrations on an inanimate object—instead of, say, your boss.

Make like Tom Cruise. Perhaps you don't want to strip down to your Skivvies like Tom did in the movie *Risky Business.* But if you can manage some privacy, crank up your favorite rock songs and play some vicious "air guitar" while dancing around like a whirling dervish. "A short dose of rock and roll and jumping around might be useful stress therapy for some people," Dr. Halpern says. Lock your office door or go down in the basement. Then pretend you're on stage with the Stones at Madison Square Garden. You'll have some fun, get rid of some nervous energy, and find yourself a lot less stressed and tense, Dr. Halpern says.

Schedule music time. Stress builds up as the day goes on. One way to keep stress from reaching unmanageable proportions is to take a scheduled "de-stress" music break each day. By taking this quick break, you'll be able to reduce some of the stress that's already built up, so you'll be better able to handle what added stress may be lurking throughout the day. "Allow yourself a bit of relaxation with music every day, even if it is only five minutes," says Dr. Halpern. Go somewhere private and listen to some relaxing slow music, he says.

Stress Training

You have weight training, strength training, aerobic training, and specialized things like marathon or bicycle race training. Now you have to pencil in stress training in your workout schedule.

According to Dr. Nicholas Hall of the Institute for Health and Human Performance, your body reacts to stress much the same way it reacts to exercise: Your heart rate and breathing increase, and you produce certain chemicals that rev up the nervous system. By using exercise, you can train the body to deal with stress and to quickly rebound from a stressful incident.

The key to Dr. Hall's stress-training exercise program is to spend most of your time working out at 70 to 80 percent of your maximum heart rate (to find your approximate maximum heart rate, subtract your age from 220) and then to rapidly increase and decrease your heart rate. You stay within that heart rate zone (the 70 to 80 percent range) for about 10 minutes. Then quickly increase your intensity until you reach 90 percent of your maximum heart rate.

Then close your eyes and relax. "The right music can automatically calm you down by relaxing your body and mind, and can slow down your heart rate and brain waves, as well."

Buy a babbling brook. A nice ocean-front property or a little cottage by a stream will do wonders for anyone's stress levels. But since most people can't afford their own luxury properties, simulated brook and ocean sounds will have to do. Nature's sounds can be very relaxing, Dr. Halpern says. "Use whatever natural sound makes you feel comfortable." You can buy tapes with the sounds of ocean waves or babbling brooks. Some plug-in machines the size of clock radios emit a variety of preprogrammed sounds

"You are putting a physical stress on the body that is somewhat similar to what your body goes through during other stress," Dr. Hall says. As soon as you hit 90 percent, slow down to about 60 percent of your target heart rate. By cutting back to 60 percent, your heart rate and breathing will slow down. "You are teaching your body how to respond to stress by recovering," he says.

After spending an amount of time at 60 percent equal to what you spent at 90 percent, go back up to the 70 to 80 percent range. Repeat this two or three times during your workout, says Dr. Hall. "By doing this exercise a few times a week, you teach your body how to come down off a stressor quickly," he says.

"In order to recover from stress, you have to first experience it. Exercise is a good stressor because it is one you can control," Dr. Hall adds. Keep in mind that you should always consult your doctor before starting any new exercise program. "It is even more important to see your doctor if you don't exercise. A lack of exercise can be more damaging to your health," he notes.

like waves, crickets in the night, or even the womblike sound of a heartbeat.

Stressing Your Skills

Like most abilities we've learned in life, reducing stress is a developed skill that gets better the more you do it. By practicing stress reduction, not only can you recover from stress faster but also you keep stress from building up in the first place. "Make relaxing a habit. It will prevent you from getting all tense and stressed out," says Dr. Larry J. Feldman of the Pain and Stress Rehabilitation Center.

If you take a few minutes every day—regardless of whether you need it—to practice stress-reduction exercises, you'll be able to reduce stress quickly when crunch time really comes around. The following can get you started on your daily de-stress routine.

Hold your breath. Just the act of breathing slowly allows you to let go of some stress, says Dennis C. Turk, Ph.D., John and Emma Bonica professor of anesthesiology and pain research at the University of Washington School of Medicine in Seattle. Sit in a comfortable place and focus on your breathing. Slowly inhale, then hold the breath for a moment. Exhale as if you are blowing on a candle but don't want to blow it out. As you repeat this, picture or mutter the word *calm* (or any word that you choose) over and over. Keep this up until you feel relaxed and calm again, Dr. Turk says.

Remind yourself. During a hectic day, it's easy to forget to take a moment to relax and keep stress in check. So that you don't forget, write "relax" with colored markers on those little yellow sticky notes and stick them in various visible places around your home or office. "When you see the signs, take a moment to relax or remind yourself of reasons that you should be happy," Dr. Feldman says. Have fun making the notes and looking at them. That will make you more likely to relax when you see them. As you look at the sticky note, take a deep breath and say the word *relax* as you exhale.

Set up a signal. Another way to remind yourself to take a quick stress break is to set up a signal. Pick something that happens a few times a day, such as the phone ringing. Then every time your phone rings, inhale, exhale as you reach for it, and say the word *relax*. "The good thing about this exercise is that it takes no time at all. If you don't have time to meditate, this will do," Dr. Feldman says.

Turning Back the Clock

Keeping Body, Mind, and Spirit Young

You can't stop the clock, go back in time, or lengthen the years. But age is only a number. You don't have to measure your youth and vitality by your chronological age. Measure it in how young you look and feel—something you can control, in other words—because even though you can't stop time, you can lessen the effects commonly associated with aging.

Younger from the Inside Out

Much of aging is linked to what you put into your body. What you consume affects how old you feel, how old you look, and how free you are of the diseases that can come with age. If you want to look and appear younger on the outside, you'll have to start from within.

Drink up. The first step to staying and feeling younger is simple: Drink water—at least six, eight-ounce glasses of filtered water per day, ideally eight if you can. "Most people are in a dehydrated phase. They should be feeling like a grape; instead, they feel like a raisin," says Chris D. Meletis, N.D., a naturopathic physician and professor of natural pharmacology and nutrition at the National College of Naturopathic Medicine in Portland, Oregon. Older folks who don't get enough water often feel irritable and have a harder time with memory.

Chuck the deep fryer. If you eat mostly fat, you'll also be heavier and less mobile in your later years. A high-fat diet also hurts your skin, Dr. Meletis says. "It makes the cell membranes more rigid. It takes the flexibility away from the skin," he says. Keep your fat intake to below 30 percent of your total calories, and limit your saturated fats.

E-asy does it. Try to get 400 international units of vitamin E a day, advises Dr. Meletis. It is hard to get that amount, or even the recommended Daily Value of 30 international units, from food, so you should take a supplement to increase your vitamin E intake. Some good food sources of vitamin E are nuts, vegetable oils, sunflower seeds, whole grains, spinach, and wheat germ.

Caution: Before taking amounts above 200 international units, discuss this with your doctor first. One study using low-dose vitamin E supplements showed an increased risk of hemorrhagic stroke.

Vitamin E is an antioxidant, which means that it can neutralize body-damaging particles called free radicals. Besides making the body more susceptible to disease, free radicals also can make you age prematurely.

C yourself younger. Vitamin C is another age-blocking antioxidant and one you'd do well to supplement in your diet. About 500 milligrams a day should help keep free radicals in check, Dr. Meletis says. Foods high in vitamin C are pineapple, pink grapefruit, oranges, kiwifruit, hot peppers, strawberries, cantaloupe, and broccoli. Your skin needs vitamin C as well, he adds. Vitamin C helps the body create collagen, which you need for healthy bones, joints, and especially skin.

Extract some help. Take 30 to 60 milligrams a day of grape seed extract, Dr. Meletis recommends. This herbal extract protects you from free radicals in two ways. First, the extract is an antioxidant itself, and protects you from free radicals. Second, the extract aids vitamins C and E, making them more powerful against free radicals, Dr. Meletis says. You'll find grape seed extract in the health food store.

Flax yourself. To moisturize your skin, which helps keep it supple and wrinkle-free, take a tablespoon of flaxseed oil every day. Or if you find the oil hard to swallow, you can take about 9,000 milligrams a day in capsule form, says Dr. Meletis. Flaxseed oil is loaded with essential fatty acids, which moisturize the skin from the inside out, keeping it bright and healthy.

Boost your brain and bravado. The two things that'll keep you feeling young no matter what are a good memory and a good sex life. Ginkgo biloba helps with both. The herb dilates blood vessels, meaning that more blood can reach both the brain and the penis, enhancing the performance of both. Like vitamins C and E, ginkgo also acts as an antioxidant, Dr. Meletis says. Buy a standardized preparation that contains 24 percent flavonoid glycosides and 6 percent ginkgolides. The typical recommended dose is one 40-milligram tablet three times daily, he says.

Caution: Taking too much concentrated ginkgo extract (more than 240 milligrams) can cause dermatitis, diarrhea, and vomiting. Also, the herb may increase the action of monoamine oxidase (MAO) inhibitors, such as Nardil, sometimes prescribed for depression.

Revitalize with ginseng. If you don't feel like you have that spring in your step like you used to, try two 100-milligram capsules of ginseng every day, says Dr. Meletis. "It's a pick-me-upper, basically." To make sure that you are getting the real thing, buy American or Siberian ginseng. Korean ginseng is not recommended, because there is a risk of it raising

---

Saving Face

Almost daily, men walk into the bathroom and perform the single best skin-care ritual ever invented.

"Men shave every day, so they are getting rid of old dead skin every single day. That's why they look younger for a long time," says Pratima Raichur, N.D., a naturopathic physician, founder of the Tej Ayurvedic Skin Care Clinic in New York City, and author of *Absolute Beauty*.

Shaving, beyond its obvious purpose, is purely a form of exfoliation. The razor scrapes off the dead layer of skin cells, exposing brighter, healthier skin. By shaving off these cells, men also help prevent the formation of wrinkles, Dr. Raichur says. Women spend a good chunk of change buying all sorts of exfoliating products: skin peels, alpha hydroxy acids, buff puffs, and loofahs. All the while, men have just been doing it with a razor—and not even knowing it.

---

blood pressure in some people. It should be standardized and contain between 4 and 7 percent ginsenosides, the active ingredient. Some ginseng products have little or no active ginsenosides, so be sure to look for the percentages on the labels. Dr. Meletis recommends taking the herb in the morning. Taking it at night could give you a boost of energy that you don't need before bedtime.

Caution: If you have high blood pressure, check with your doctor before taking ginseng.

Going with the Flow

Blood acts as a transit system for your body. With regular deliveries of oxygen and other nutrients, your bloodstream keeps your brain going, your skin healthy, and your organs functioning.

The ancient arts of acupressure and yoga focus on keeping the blood pumping all throughout your body. Take a few minutes each day to practice the following to make you feel and look younger.

Take a stretch break. "Participating regularly in stretching regimens like yoga keeps your body young internally and externally," says yoga instructor Mara Carrico. Yoga poses and breathing exercises increase circulation and enhance the functioning of all organs, including your skin. Here is one exercise to try that can help you keep feeling young.

Lie on your back with your legs up a wall. Your buttocks should be six to eight inches from the wall, and your legs relaxed and six inches apart. Place a folded towel under your neck so that your head and neck are supported and your face is parallel to the ceiling. Keep your arms at your sides. Close your eyes and hold this pose for three to five minutes.

Caution: Check with your doctor first if you have hypertension or glaucoma.

Rub your ears. Massage your ears lightly every day for at least two minutes. During the massage, lightly pull the ear, especially the earlobe, in various directions. This will increase circulation and could have an impact on longevity, believes Dr. Michael Reed Gach of the Acupressure Institute.

Only Skin-Deep

Women don't have a lock on the skin-care market. Wrinkles make men look just as old, and maybe more gnarly. You want to look good as you get older, not just, well, older.

Although a market has erupted that encourages chemically peeling off your face and injecting yourself with synthetic substances, nature has given you a variety of options to keep your skin healthy and young looking for a long time.

Clean yourself up. The first step in great skin is to cleanse your face, says Dr. Pratima Raichur of the Tej Ayurvedic Skin Care Clinic. Cleansing removes the dead cells and toxins that take hold of the skin. Apply some face soap or facial cleanser before shaving. Massage it into your skin and then wash it off with warm water.

Buy a cleanser that pertains to your skin type—oily, sensitive, or dry. Make sure that it only contains natural ingredients—no synthetic substances, no mineral oils, no chemicals, no dyes, no preservatives, and no fragrances.

Use an essential aftershave. After you shave, apply essential oils to your skin instead of aftershave, Dr. Raichur advises. Although aftershave keeps razor burns and cuts from getting infected, the alcohol content burns and hurts the skin. Pour two ounces of water into a spray bottle and add 10 drops of your favorite essential oil (lemon, sandalwood, and sweet orange are good ones for men). Spritz this solution on your face as a refreshing aftershave, Dr. Raichur recommends.

If you experience redness or irritation, rinse the area with cold water, cut the concentration in half, or don't use the oils at all.

Moisturize your mug. The last step in the Ayurvedic skin-care routine is moisturizing your face, Dr. Raichur says. "You can use any kind of moisturizing cream, but it is always good to use an herbal one," she says. You'll find herbal creams in health food stores or herb stores. Make sure that the one you select has all-natural ingredients.

Break open some E. Applying vitamin E directly to the skin softens wrinkles and crow's feet, Dr. Meletis says. Break open a vitamin E capsule and rub the gel-like vitamin into wrinkled areas of your skin. You can do this once a day or as needed, he says.

Comfort with calendula. The herb calendula is often used as an antiseptic for cuts. But Dr. Meletis says that cream made with calendula can also do wonders for your skin. The herb helps heal skin tissue, making your skin look healthier, he says. Calendula herbal cream works well whether used every day or just as needed, he says.

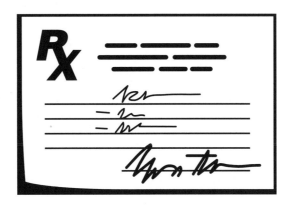

Part Four

Natural Cures

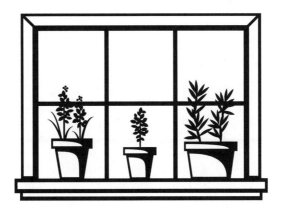

The Natural Medicine Chest

Prepare for Healing

Drive past any strip mall and you'll likely see 24-hour drugstores, supermarkets, and convenience stores. Just who are they open for? Who goes shopping at 3:30 A.M. on a Wednesday?

Probably you do. You and the rest of the population who wake up with relentless coughs and blazing fevers only to find that your medicine cabinets contain shaving cream and two-year-old aspirin. No one wants or intends to be in a store during the graveyard shift. But many a man has found himself dressed in a T-shirt and sweatpants in the cold and flu aisle at 4:00 A.M. It often seems like whatever remedy you really need at the moment, you won't have on hand.

But a little forward thinking and a shopping list can turn your home into an alternative medicine triage center ready for many ailments. The following is a list of natural and alternative remedies for your basic everyday health problems. These are the majority of the natural ingredients that you will need to heed the advice in the following chapters. Stock up your home with these, and you'll never find yourself shopping with the living dead again.

Herbs and Plants

It's hard to consider herbal remedies all that alternative when you can buy them at your local supermarket or chain drugstore. Although many stores now carry the following recommended herbs—some even in the produce section—you may want to start your search in a health food store or a store that specializes in herbs, says James A. Duke, Ph.D., a botanist retired from the U.S. Department of Agriculture and author of *The Green Pharmacy.* These stores are likely to know more about herbs and reputable herbal companies.

Aloe vera plant. The best way to ensure you get quality aloe is to buy an aloe plant. Use it for burns and bruises.

Arnica montana. This homeopathic herb is used for healing bruises.

Calendula. Calendula is a natural antiseptic used for cuts and bruises.

Echinacea. This herb is used for colds or the flu. It activates white blood cells that kill cold viruses. It can also be used to prevent infection of a cut or scrape.

Garlic. Garlic helps kill cold-causing viruses and other bacteria. Also, garlic has been shown to lower cholesterol and improve heart health.

Ginseng. This overall tonic is taken as a pick-me-up. Use during times of poor energy.

Parsley. Have homemade parsley ice cubes on hand for bruises. Parsley helps bruises heal faster.

Tea tree oil. Use this oil for colds, asthma, and allergy attacks. It also works as an antiseptic for skin problems, cuts, and scrapes.

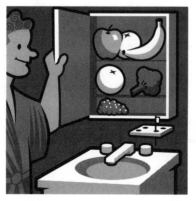

Teas

Easy to make and easy to take, teas are wonderful ways to use herbal medicines. In some ways, you get more of the healing properties of an herb in tea form. You mostly use dried herbs to make herbal tea. Because dried herbs have less water content than fresh herbs, the less volatile active ingredients become more concentrated. So teas made of dried herbs can sometimes be more potent than fresh herb concoctions, says Dr. Duke. When you add the water, more of the active ingredients are infused in the tea, increasing its power. If you only have fresh herbs on hand, you need to use four times as much of the herb to get the same potency, he says.

But remember that once an herb is harvested, its potency decreases the longer you store it. So use the herb as soon as possible after harvesting, says Dr. Duke.

Many of the following teas can be found in already-made tea bags at supermarkets or health food stores. For others, you may have to buy dried herbs and make your own tea—called an infusion, in herbal jargon. Place a teaspoon of the dried herb in boiling water and steep it for 10 minutes, says Dr. Duke. If you are really industrious, you can make your own tea bag by placing a teaspoon of the herb in muslin—a lightweight cotton fabric. Use it as you would a regular tea bag, he says.

Chamomile. Chamomile tea quiets the stomach and the mind. Use it for general stomach upset. It is also a good relaxant during times of stress.

Ginger. Ginger tea helps quell a nauseated stomach and is also good for motion sickness.

Licorice root tea with marshmallow. This tea calms colitis and other digestive inflammation problems. Or use geranium, slippery elm bark, goldenseal, or yarrow teas.

Peppermint, spearmint, or blackberry. These teas help soothe upset stomachs.

Stinging nettle. This herb works as an antihistamine and calms allergies.

Willow bark. This herb works as a pain reliever, reduces fever, and is also an anti-inflammatory.

Nature's Bandage

A poultice is a wad of chopped plant material that you apply directly to a wound or skin infection. You usually keep it in place with a wet dressing covered by a bandage. All you really need to make a poultice is the herb or plant matter and something to keep it in place. Take the herb or plant and pound it until it is pulverized. Then mold it into a coin-size wad. Lay it flat against the wound, and then use gauze or clothing to keep the plant in place over the wound.

Poultices work directly on the wound or infection, but many of the healing compounds probably pass through the skin and help you internally. You could also make a poultice by boiling or steaming the herb, mixing it with three parts water, alcohol, or vinegar, and then thickening it with flour.

Essential Oils

Essential oils help with a wide variety of ailments, says Michael Scholes of the Michael Scholes School of Aromatic Studies. Essential oils provide the basis of aromatherapy—the treatment of medical problems with aromatic essential oils of fragrant herbs. The oils usually come in small vials and are extremely concentrated. If diluted properly, many can be used in massage, added to grooming products, and dropped into baths. A variety of aromatherapy products such as diffusers and candles help emit the smells and healing qualities of essential oils. Essential oils should only be used externally. Most are toxic if ingested.

Although there are thousands of different oils, start with the following ones, Scholes recommends. It's not easy to figure out if you are getting a good product, he warns. Essential oil products used to be limited to a select group of suppliers and health stores but now can be found in retail stores and malls. He recommends looking for a toll-free number or a company address on the product. That way, if you have questions, you have someone whom you can ask for help, he says.

Eucalyptus. In combination with peppermint and tea tree oils, eucalyptus is used for asthma and allergy attacks.

Lavender. Lavender acts as an anti-inflammatory and is good for digestive muscle spasms, back pain, or other sore, inflamed muscles. It is also used for headaches.

Peppermint. This essential oil is used for many ailments such as colds, allergies, or asthma. Combined with birch and wintergreen, it can be used for back pain.

Rosemary and juniper. Used in conjunction with peppermint, they're good for a stuffy head and blocked sinuses.

Tree oils. Different from tea tree oil, these oils of fir, pine, and myrtle help respiration during a cold or allergy or asthma attack.

Nutrition

Although the actual science of nutrition has only been around for the last quarter-century or so, the use of nutrition as a healing mechanism has been around for ages. Years ago, people used food and nutrition to cure all kinds of diseases. Experts have concluded that proper nutrition could cut death rates from cardiovascular diseases, infection and respiratory diseases, cancer, and diabetes. ·

Beyond the major diseases that can be helped by nutrition, some of your common everyday problems benefit from having a few food staples around the house. Stock up on the following foods, vitamins, and minerals, and you'll be set to fight off a good deal of ailments the old-fashioned way.

Fruits and vegetables. Fruits and vegetables may provide the basis of every immune-boosting diet. Citrus fruits high in vitamin C are good for colds and can help bruises heal faster.

Psyllium. This natural form of soluble fiber helps with both diarrhea and constipation.

Salt. Keep a jar of salt in your medicine cabinet to help with sore throats.

Vitamin B$_6$. Vitamin B$_6$ is essential for proper brain and nerve function.

Vitamin C. This nutrient is used for general good health, fighting off colds, and decreasing seasonal allergies. It can also help heal cuts and bruises.

Vitamin E. This vitamin reduces heart disease risk and prevents heart attacks.

Zinc lozenges. Zinc lozenges may help reduce the duration of a cold.

Tools of the Trade

Having the right materials around is only half the battle in building a natural medicine chest. A few tools are needed to help make some of the remedies, or at least make them easier to use. Have a few of the following on hand so that you're completely prepared for your next at-home health crisis, says aromatherapist and herbalist Jeanne Rose, executive director of the Aromatic Plant Project, a nonprofit organization based in San Francisco, and author of *The World of Aromatherapy*.

- A strainer. After steeping herbs in a tea, you'll need something to fish them out before you can drink it. Your basic kitchen strainer or a piece of cheesecloth will do the trick.
- Eyedroppers. Use separate droppers for taking tinctures and using essential oils.
- Candles. Buy special candles that already have essential oils in them.
- Porcelain or glass diffusers. They allow the essential oils to volatilize and diffuse into the atmosphere. Some can be plugged in or are made of pottery.

Boosting Your Immunity

Building a Strong Defense

Your immune system is smart. Throughout evolution, it has learned to detect the millions of outside invaders that try to find their way into your body. It knows what should be there, what shouldn't, and how to get rid of unwelcome visitors. The complex line of defense starts with your skin, the first barrier for attackers to cross. It has secondary defenses: nose hair, mucus, and saliva. If anything gets past all of that, your immune system turns to chemical warfare to destroy the invader once and for all.

Despite all its accumulated knowledge, your immune system is not fail-proof. Like any other complex machine, it needs to be taken care of to perform at its best. That's where you come in. By taking the right steps, you can ensure that it's ready at all times to do its job.

Feeding the Army

There's no magic fruit or vegetable that will make you a virtual man of steel when it comes to your immunity. But when you stop to think about it, that's actually good news. Mother Nature gives us products that contain a wealth of substances to maintain a strong immune system. Every fruit and vegetable packs powerful yet different immunity-enhancing chemicals, nutrients, and a host

of other things that science hasn't even discovered yet. Instead of relying on one or two select fruits, you can pick from all of them and know that you've just done something to help maintain a healthy immune system.

To use food to strengthen your immunity, you must eat a wide variety of fruits, vegetables, and whole grains, says Thomas Petro, Ph.D., associate professor of microbiology and immunology at the University of Nebraska Medical Center in Lincoln. By casting a wide net, you're bound to hit many of the nutrients found in food that build up your natural defense system. By sticking to only a select group, you're missing out on many of the nutrients you need.

Unlike supplements, food delivers these immune-enhancing nutrients in the best package. We know from studies that people who eat fruits and vegetables have better immune systems. But many times, a researcher will extract a particular vitamin or nutrient from a food, thinking that it's the key to the fruit or vegetable's power. But when the tests come in, it often doesn't show the same beneficial results. It may be that only the natural form of the nutrient works. It may be that another nutrient present in the food is responsible. Or it could be that it isn't one nutrient but how all the nutrients work together that keeps an immune system healthy. "We simply don't know enough about them yet," says Susanna Cunningham-Rundles, Ph.D., associate professor of immunology at New York Hospital–Cornell Medical Center in New York City.

So your best bet is to eat at least five—and preferably closer to nine—servings of fruits and vegetables a day, eat whole grains, and cut down on fat. "For the guy seeking to keep his immune system strong and healthy, you have to start with the basics," says acupuncturist Victor S. Sierpina, M.D., assistant professor of family medicine at the University of Texas Medical Branch in Galveston.

Covering All the Bases

Although no one denies that the best way to get the nutrients you need is through food, there are a few standout vitamins and minerals. These few have proved to be integral to the functioning of the immune system. Without them, your defense system has a gaping hole in it.

Vitamin E. Take a supplement of 400 international units of vitamin E a day, says Dr. Petro. Because it is found mainly in fat, it is hard to get the amount of vitamin E you need for a healthy immune system. If you are considering taking vitamin E in amounts above 200 international units, discuss this with your doctor first. One study using low-dose vitamin E supplements showed an increased risk of hemorrhagic stroke.

Vitamin E acts as an antioxidant, protecting your body from disease-causing molecules called free radicals. Studies have shown that extra vitamin E enhances the immune function in animals and people. "The most astonishing results we have seen are with vitamin E," Dr. Petro says. A study at Tufts University in Boston found that having older people supplement with vitamin E improved their immune systems.

Vitamin C. You should take a supplement of 500 milligrams a day of vitamin C. "Vitamin C is a factor in normal immune cells," says Dennis D. Taub, Ph.D., acting chief of the laboratory of immunology at the National Institute on Aging in Baltimore. Numerous studies have shown that vitamin C is needed for a healthy immune system. Like vitamin E, vitamin C is an antioxidant and prevents disease by controlling free radicals. Some studies have even linked vitamin C to fighting off infections.

Zinc. Without zinc, many of the immune cells can't do their job. This trace mineral is critical for immune function. Yet a little goes a long way with zinc. Stick to the Daily Value of 15 milligrams, about what you will find in a multivitamin/mineral, says Chris D. Meletis, N.D., a naturopathic physician and professor of natural pharmacology and nutrition at the National College of Naturopathic Medicine in Portland, Oregon. Too much zinc actually suppresses your immune system because of the depletion of copper.

B vitamins. Three of the important B vitamins—B_6, B_{12}, and folic acid—play major roles in keeping your immune system up and running. You deplete your B vitamins during times of stress, says Dr. Sierpina. So it is important to get them either in a multivitamin or in a B-complex supplement. Look for the Daily Value of all three: 2 milligrams of vitamin B_6, 6 micrograms of B_{12}, and 400 micrograms of folic acid. Someone under a lot of stress should try to get even higher amounts of B vitamins, says Dr. Sierpina.

Passing the Stress Test

Nothing can shut down your immune system like stress. "Stress has incredible effects on the immune system. It is monstrous," Dr. Taub says. When your body goes into its fight-or-flight mode, it saps all the energy from your natural defense system, leaving you more open to all kinds of nasty things. So control stress, and you'll gain some control over your immune system's health. Here are some ways suggested by experts.

Listen to the music. The right music can aid you in your quest for calm in a stressed-out world, says Steven Halpern, Ph.D., president of Inner Peace Music in San Anselmo, California, and a composer. "It's like vitamins in the airwaves. You can enhance your immunity by choosing music that evokes your relaxation response," he says. There are several ways that you can use music to decrease your stress and help your immune system.

• Keep headphones in your office. Having instrumental, light music in the background creates a calming atmosphere in your office. If playing music in the background disturbs co-workers and you can work with headphones on, do so, Dr. Halpern says. If the music distracts you, use the headphones to take stress breaks. Instead of a coffee break, use those 5 to 10 minutes to take a music break. Put the headphones on and relax, he says.

• Move to the music. Call in the rock-'n'-roll doctor. Put on whatever music makes you get up and dance. Sing, play "air guitar," or prance around the room to a song to which you can rock out. Do this for 10 minutes, and you'll get out some aggression and have some fun, Dr. Halpern says.

• Pick up sticks. You don't have to buy a drum. A pencil and your desk will do just fine. Rap on your desk. The physical act of making rhythmic music releases some pent-up frustration and tension, Dr. Halpern says.

Take a breather. A simple breathing exercise can restore some peace to a crazed day, says Larry J. Feldman, Ph.D., director of the Pain and Stress Rehabilitation Center in New Castle, Delaware, and author of *Feeling Good Again*, a self-help book for dealing with stress. This breathing technique should help you relax, get some sleep, if need be, and provide control over tension: Inhale. When your lungs feel full, exhale naturally. After you have exhaled naturally, push out even more air for a count of 10. Start all over again by inhaling. Repeat the process five times, he says.

If you need to chill out some more, take

Eat Less, Live Longer

The secret to a long life and better immunity may lie in how much you eat as well as in what you eat.

It has been shown that eating less slows the rate of aging," says George Roth, Ph.D., a researcher at the gerontology research center at the National Institute on Aging in Baltimore. If you slow the aging rate, you also improve immunity since immune function decreases with age.

Researchers aren't sure why restricting calories keeps you and your immunity young. One theory is that your metabolism works better with less food. But no one is ready to tell people to stop eating. Dr. Roth says that he and his researchers haven't come up with a set number of calories and that it could be different for each person. He also worries about people developing nutrient deficiencies, which could cause serious health problems. "We are not ready to recommend it," he says.

Another researcher adds that most studies have been done with mice, and it's difficult to transfer those results into people terms. "Humans are more difficult to study. With mice, we don't have to worry about ice cream," says Dr. Dennis D. Taub of the National Institute on Aging.

a two-minute break, then do the exercise five more times. To really control stress, practice this once or twice a day. By making it a habit, you'll stay calm during times of stress, Dr. Feldman says. If you are short on time, simply focus your attention on your breathing.

Count backward. When all you see is red, take a moment and start counting backward from the number 40. With each number, take a full breath. In your mind, count each breath off as you exhale, saying the word *relax* after each number you count. By the time you reach zero, you should be in more control, Dr. Feldman says. Not only will this work in the heat of a stressful situation but also it will do wonders if you practice it once a day. "It will prevent you from getting all tense and stressed out. The more you do it, the better it will work. And in no time, you won't need to count back from 40," Dr. Feldman says. Practice enough, and you'll be able to get the same calming effect counting from 20, or even lower, he says.

Rub out stress. A good massage not only reduces stress but also has actually been shown to boost immunity on its own. A study at the University of Miami School of Medicine found that men who were HIV-positive and who received daily massages for a month saw a jump in the number of their natural killer cells—cells that protect you from diseases. "When a person is touched and massaged in a therapeutic manner, the body's system is going to react," says Robert A. Edwards, a licensed massage therapist and director of the Somerset School of Massage Therapy in New Jersey. Do some at-home massage, or make an appointment with a qualified massage therapist.

Sign up for yoga. Yoga postures and breathing techniques, if practiced regularly, bring about a serenity that lingers with you throughout the day. "A yoga workout generally relieves stress," says Mara Carrico, a yoga instructor based in San Diego, creator of *The 10-Minute Yoga Work-In* audiocassette program, and author of *Yoga Journal's Yoga Basics.* Many yoga classes or workouts end with a meditation. Meditation helps you let go of stress and can add to the quality of your life by teaching you how to live each moment to the fullest, Carrico says.

Meet the Press

According to the Chinese technique of acupressure, all the stress you encounter creates an energy imbalance in your body. This imbalance then weakens your immune system. Several acupressure points are believed to get that energy back on track and bring back balance and a healthier immunity.

Lend an ear. Place your finger on the piece of cartilage that is in front of your ear canal. Put your thumb behind this piece of your ear cartilage and squeeze. For best results, pinch hard enough so that you feel a hot stinging sensation. This point, called the adrenal point, stimulates hormone production to kick-start your immunity, says David Nickel, a doctor of Oriental medicine; a certified acupuncturist in Santa Monica, California; and author of *Acupressure for Athletes.* Squeeze the point for five seconds as you exhale through your mouth, then let up for five seconds as you inhale through your nose. Continue these five-second intervals for about a minute.

Reach for your funny bone. An acupressure point in the elbow crease, called the Crooked Pond, is thought to correct weaknesses in the immune system. Bend your arm so that you form a crease inside your elbow. Place your thumb on the upper edge of the crease on the outside of your arm. Apply firm pressure into the joint and hold for one minute as you breathe deeply. Do this twice a day, says Michael Reed Gach, Ph.D., founder of the Acupressure Institute in Berkeley, California, and author of *Acupressure's Potent Points.*

"You should feel a slight pain, but it will be a good hurt," Dr. Gach says.

Unleash your energy. Get on your back with your knees bent to activate this point, which strengthens the immune system, Dr. Gach says. The point, called the Sea of Energy, is two finger-widths below the belly button, between the belly button and the pubic bone. Apply firm pressure down and in toward the vertebrae in your lower back. You know that you have the correct point if you feel the pressure deep inside, Dr. Gach says. Breathe deeply as you hold the point for two minutes.

Nature's Reinforcements

Several herbs are believed to have immune-boosting qualities. Now that herbs have experienced a renaissance of sorts, you should be able to find the following in drugstores, supermarkets, or health food stores.

Derail the cold bug. Echinacea acts as an immunostimulant. Simply put, it rallies your immune system. By doing so, it increases your body's resistance to bacterial invaders. Take it in a tea or tincture form since there is some indication that it activates the immune system through mucosal absorption in the mouth. Take it at the first sign of a cold or flu. You can also take it if you have been exposed to someone with a cold, like that co-worker who came in and sneezed all over your office, says Dr. Meletis. "It may help abort the cold from taking you over," he says.

To make a tea from echinacea, pour boiling water over two to three tablespoons of dried, fresh, or powdered herb and steep for five minutes. Drink three cups a day. Or take 30 drops of tincture three times a day. Double this dosage if you want to ease the symptoms two or three days after the onset of a cold, Dr. Meletis says.

Do not use echinacea for more than eight weeks at a time; if you have an autoimmune condition such as lupus, tuberculosis, or multiple sclerosis; or if you are allergic to chamomile, marigold, or other plants in the daisy family.

Ward off diseases with garlic. In olden times, some people claimed that garlic could cure "all diseases." That may be overstating it, but garlic is a talented herb/food when it comes to immunity. Garlic has been shown to lower cholesterol and thin the blood, which could help prevent heart attacks and strokes. It appears to block the growth of cancer cells. And it has been shown to kill at least 14 strains of bacteria taken from the noses and throats of children.

The best way to get garlic is to toss about a clove a day in with your cooking, Dr. Meletis says. If you dislike the pungent aroma of fresh garlic, you can take enteric-coated capsules. Take enough garlic to get 4,000 micrograms of allicin a day.

Go for an oil change. The essential oils thyme, peppermint, and pine increase your body's energy and boost your body's natural defense system, says Michael Scholes, president and founder of the Michael Scholes School of Aromatic Studies in Los Angeles. You can use each of the oils separately or mix a combination of them together, depending on your personal preference, he says. Try a massage with them, heavily diluting them in carrier oils such as canola, jojoba, or sweet almond, he says. Using 10 to 12 drops of essential oil in an ounce of massage oil is just right. Any scent that makes you feel good reduces stress, which, in turn, can help your immune system, Scholes adds. But be aware that some essential oils can cause skin irritation or may even be toxic. Check with a knowledgeable aromatherapist before experimenting with them.

A Little Help from Your Friends

Hanging out with family and friends is good for your health.

Researchers at Carnegie Mellon University in Pittsburgh took 276 healthy people and injected them with a common cold virus. They were also asked about their relationships with spouses, parents, friends, workmates, and social groups. Those with the most types of social interactions were less likely to develop the common cold. They even produced less mucus if they did catch the cold. Those with fewer social outlets had greater chances of getting sick.

Heart Disease

*Knocking a Killer
out of the Top Spot*

It has been at the top of the charts almost every year since 1900, but it's not something that Casey Kasem would be proud to announce every week. Heart disease has had a lock on the number one spot as a killer of Americans for most of the past century, and it looks as if it will keep that position well into the next millennium. More than 2,600 Americans die each day from cardiovascular diseases—about one every 33 seconds.

But heart disease doesn't just happen to you. You don't catch it like a cold. It takes time to develop. That gives you a number of chances to jump in and stop it from happening, or least lessen some of its effects. And it's never too late to start fighting. A number of simple, natural techniques—stress reduction, diet, supplements, even the music you listen to—can give you the upper hand against this killer.

From the Outside In

Heart disease is clearly related to what you put in your mouth, though it has many other important causes, as well. By the same token, what passes your lips can also protect you from this disease. The key is to strike a perfect balance between getting the good things to end up in your stomach and keeping the not-so-good ones out.

Get high on fiber. Don't peel that apple, and by all means finish off that potato,

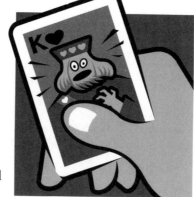

skin and all. Fruits and vegetable skins are filled with fiber, especially a fiber called pectin. Pectin grabs hold of cholesterol floating around your body and takes it out of your system, where it can't damage your arteries or heart. Other ways to fill up on fiber include choosing whole-grain cereals and breads, substituting beans for meat in your taco, and peeling the skin off citrus fruits and eating them whole—don't cut them. The white stringy stuff on the outside of the fruit is pectin, too. Beans and lentils pack a powerful fiber punch, and soy also helps fight heart disease. Before you know it, you'll be up to the recommended 25 grams of fiber a day, says Dr. Victor S. Sierpina of the University of Texas Medical Branch.

Weed out the fat. Say goodbye to the deep fryer. Look for cuts of beef such as tip round, bottom round, and top sirloin in the butcher store. Substitute marinades and chicken broth for oils and grease. Search nutrition labels for fat content, and make sure that it is less than 30 percent of the total calories. All of these moves will cut out some fat in your life, which, in turn, will be good for your heart, says Dr. Sierpina.

Fight for your phytochemicals. With every meal, you should have one or two servings of a fruit or a vegetable. It's not that hard. Slice a banana on top of your cereal and have a glass of orange juice for breakfast. Have a salad with lunch and an apple for dessert. For dinner, grill up some zucchini, peppers, and mushrooms and make them the focus of dinner. Following that standard, you'll be up to five or more servings a day of fruits and vegetables before you know it. By doing so, you ensure getting a wealth of phytochemicals that protect against heart disease, says Robert Cullen, R.D., Ph.D., assistant professor of food and nutrition, and nutrition and dietetics program director at Illinois State University in Normal.

Find more folic acid. Get 400 micrograms of folic acid a day—the recommended Daily Value and an amount usually found in a typical multivitamin. Folate—the natural form of folic acid, found in food—depresses an amino acid in your body called homocysteine, says John N. Hathcock, Ph.D., director of nutrition and regulatory science for the Council for Responsible Nutrition in Washington, D.C. The more homocysteine you have in your system, the more likely you are to develop heart disease. You can get folate from foods such as orange juice and green leafy vegetables. But your body better absorbs folic acid from a multivitamin than it does folate from food, Dr. Hathcock adds.

Look to the sea. Enjoy the likes of fatty fish such as tuna, salmon, mackerel, and shellfish. These fish are loaded with omega-3 fatty acids, a nutrient believed to lower the risk of heart attacks. In a study of more than 20,000 male physicians, researchers at the Women's Hospital in Boston found that those who ate fish once a week had a 52 percent lower risk of having a sudden fatal heart attack than those who didn't eat fish had. "This is probably due to the omega-3 fatty acids in fish," Dr. Sierpina says. He recommends a pesco-vegetarian (fish and vegetables) diet to those seeking to lose weight and reduce cardiac risk. Try for a serving of a high omega-3 fish three times a week.

Look to the C (and E). Dr. Sierpina himself takes vitamin C and vitamin E every day to protect himself from heart disease. "These antioxidants protect against oxidative stress and cholesterol accumulation," he says. Vitamin C is thought to do a number of things to prevent heart disease, such as reduce cholesterol, repair damaged artery walls, and prevent low-density lipoprotein (LDL, the "bad") cholesterol from oxidizing, which promotes heart disease.

In a study of more than 2,000 patients with heart disease, those who took 400 to 800

An Affair of the Heart

It seems that the Beatles were on to something when they sang, "Love is all you need." At least, that's the belief of the country's heart disease guru, Dean Ornish, M.D., president and director of the Preventive Medicine Research Institute in Sausalito, California, and author of *Dr. Dean Ornish's Program for Reversing Heart Disease.*

According to Dr. Ornish, a lack of love and intimacy in a person's life ranks up there with high cholesterol, smoking, and stress as a risk factor of heart disease.

In his book *Love and Survival,* Dr. Ornish points to several studies that show the effects of love on heart disease. At one study at Yale University School of Medicine, researchers interviewed 119 men and 40 women who were having their coronary arteries x-rayed to see the extent of blockages. Those who said that they felt the most loved had substantially less blockage than the others had.

Another study, at Case Western Reserve University in Cleveland, focused on 10,000 married men. Even if they had risk factors such as high cholesterol and high blood pressure, men who said yes to the question "Does your wife show you her love?" had fewer chest pain attacks than the men who answered no had.

Dr. Ornish's book suggests using more positive words when you talk to others, joining support groups, practicing confession and forgiveness, and helping others through service.

international units of vitamin E reduced their risks of heart attack by 75 percent. Take 1,000 milligrams of vitamin C and 400 international units of vitamin E every day for improved health, suggests Dr. Sierpina. If you are considering taking vitamin E in amounts above 200 international units, discuss this with your doctor first. One study using low-dose vitamin E supplements showed an increased risk of hemorrhagic stroke. Excess vitamin C may cause diarrhea in some people.

Take a cue from co-Q$_{10}$. If you have a history of heart disease, or if anyone in your immediate family does, then you may want to take coenzyme Q$_{10}$ (co-Q$_{10}$). Take between 50 to 100 milligrams of the enzyme, says Shari Lieberman, Ph.D., a certified nutrition specialist, clinical nutritionist in New York City, and author of *The Real Vitamin and Mineral Book.* Capsules usually come in 10-, 30-, 50-, and 100-milligram form. Supplementing with co-Q$_{10}$ has been shown to improve the health of heart disease patients and has even allowed some patients to reduce the number and amount of heart medications they take (under a doctor's supervision, of course). When someone has a heart attack, he tends to lack co-Q$_{10}$, says Dr. Lieberman. It may also help prevent heart disease because it acts as an antioxidant, she adds.

Carry breath mints. You'll need them for when you start eating garlic. About one clove a day, either in your food or through garlic pills, may help reduce your risk for a heart attack, says Dr. Sierpina. If you are opting for the garlic capsules, check the label and make sure that your daily dose will give you at least 10 milligrams of allicin. The garlic may work in two ways: First, studies have shown that it helps keep cholesterol down; and second, garlic may also prevent blood platelets from sticking together, which decreases your odds of a heart attack, Dr. Sierpina says.

Ginkgo with the flow. The ancient herb ginkgo dilates the blood vessels, allowing blood to flow freely. "Ginkgo is beneficial for circulation in general," Dr. Sierpina says. Look

for standardized ginkgo with 24 percent flavonoid glycosides and 6 percent ginkgolides. Take one 40-milligram tablet three times daily, Dr. Sierpina suggests. The herb helps the heart in additional ways. Ginkgo helps prevent blood platelets from binding together, a condition that can provoke a heart attack in some people. Ginkgo also acts as an antioxidant, keeping LDL cholesterol from oxidizing and damaging blood vessels. But be careful. Taking too much concentrated ginkgo extract (more than 240 milligrams) can cause dermatitis, diarrhea, and vomiting. This herb may also increase the action of certain monoamine oxidase (MAO) inhibitors, such as Nardil.

Schedule tea time. Instead of brewing a pot of coffee, take the time to brew a cup of tea—even iced tea, if you prefer. Tea bags are teeming with compounds called polyphenols, says Joe A. Vinson, Ph.D., professor of chemistry at the University of Scranton in Pennsylvania.

These polyphenols act as antioxidants, keeping cholesterol from hardening and clogging up your arteries. Be sure to buy real tea, not herbal, because herbal tea doesn't have enough of the polyphenols. Look for black tea, the kind you find in regular supermarket tea bags, or green tea, which is more readily available in health food stores. As long as you use real tea bags and brew it, iced tea has the same heart disease–fighting qualities as hot tea.

Toss one back. It sounds too good to be true, but an apple schnapps a day may help keep the cardiologist away. An American Cancer Society study of 490,000 people showed that those who drank one alcoholic drink a day—be it beer, wine, or Mad Dog—reduced their risks of death by 21 percent and reduced their risks of heart disease by 30 to 40 percent. (A drink is defined as 12 ounces of beer, 5 ounces of wine, or 1½ ounces of 80-proof distilled spirits.) "Those who got the largest benefit were those at higher risk of heart disease and stroke," Michael J. Thun, M.D., study author and director of analytic epidemiology at the

American Cancer Society in Atlanta. The key word here is "moderation." Take more than one a day, and you risk shortening your life span.

If you want to get an extra punch against heart disease, make your one drink a dark beer or red wine. Those two drinks contain antioxidant polyphenols, just like tea, Dr. Vinson says. Polyphenols have been shown to keep cholesterol from oxidizing, which can prevent heart disease.

Go for the grapes. If alcohol isn't your thing, down a glass of grape juice instead. Grape juice is red wine without the alcohol, so it does contain the heart disease–fighting polyphenols, Dr. Vinson says. When buying grape juice, look at the list of ingredients. You want grape juice, not grape-flavored water with tons of sugar. Check the label for words like 100 percent pure or real grape juice, with no additives or preservatives. Grape juice should be listed on the label as the first and main ingredient, he says.

Stressful on Your Heart

Author Russell Hoban once wrote of stress: "When you suffer an attack of nerves, you're being attacked by the nervous system. What chance has a man got against a system?"

It's an accurate description of both the action and the futility you'll feel once you go into stress mode. You perceive the stress in your mind, and your body also reacts. You start to pump out chemicals called adrenaline and cortisol (often the start of what scientists call the fear response). When they hit your bloodstream, they increase your heart rate, tighten your heart muscles, and send your blood

Working Can Be Hard on the Heart

Some Mondays, people feel like death warmed over, and maybe for a good reason. More heart attacks occur on Mondays than on any other day of the week. Saturday comes in a distant second. This seems contradictory, we know. But it's thought by researchers and physicians alike that any new adjustment—whether it's to a new workweek or even a new day of leisure—can put enough stress on someone to weaken the heart.

While you consider calling in sick on Monday, you may also want to take a good look at the connection between your job and your heart health. Over and above the everyday job stress that everyone experiences, people with little control over their work have 3.8 to 4.8 times as many heart attacks as those people who have high-control jobs have, according to Adriane Fugh-Berman, M.D., former head of field investigations for the Office of Alternative Medicine at the National Institutes of Health in Bethesda, Maryland, and author of *Alternative Medicine: What Works.* Low-control jobs include cooks, waiters, cashiers, assembly line workers, nurse's aides, postal workers, and computer operators. High-control jobs are architects, barbers, civil engineers, dentists, foresters, foremen, natural scientists, programmers, sales representatives, social workers, and therapists.

Along with stress-management techniques for the prevention and treatment of heart disease, Dr. Victor S. Sierpina of the University of Texas Medical Branch may recommend a job change for some people. Dr. Sierpina also adds that having value and meaning in your work and in your life is good for your heart and soul.

pressure through the roof. Your eyes, nose, and throat all widen. Your digestive process comes to a stop. Your muscles recoil with tension. Obviously, going through this process often is not a good experience for your heart, and it also closes down your body's peripheral vascular system, which causes cold hands and feet.

A study of 901 Finnish men found that the men who had the most extreme jump in blood pressure during stress also had the thickest blockages in their carotid arteries, the blood vessels that flow blood to the brain. The strongest correlation was for men under 55. Like other risk factors such as high cholesterol, over time, stress is likely to damage blood vessels and promote hardening of the arteries in some people.

A study at Johns Hopkins University in Baltimore found that people under 60 who succumb to stress easily may have greater risks of developing heart disease. Those who developed ischemia—lack of blood flow to the heart—during exercise were 21 times more likely to have a dangerous response to mental stress.

You do have a chance when you stand against your own system, says Dr. Larry J. Feldman of the Pain and Stress Rehabilitation Center. All you need to do is learn how to handle stress, he explains.

Here are several ways to allow your body and your mind to return to a more healthful, more positive mind-body state.

Take a deep breather. Sit on a chair or lie down. Close your eyes and calmly repeat the word *relax* 40 times, counting back from 40 to 0, saying the number followed by the word *relax*. "You will feel calmer and more in control by the time you get to zero," Dr. Feldman says. After doing this exercise a few times a day, you'll find that you won't need to count back from 40. You'll be able to relax by 20, then you'll be able to get yourself into a relaxed state within a short period of time, Dr. Feldman says.

Soothe the savage blood pressure. Listen to calm, soothing music during times of stress. Certain music has been shown to bring

down blood pressure and counteract the harmful effects of stress, says Dr. Steven Halpern of Inner Peace Music. In general, most instrumental music with a slow and gentle beat should calm you down. If you need ideas, Dr. Halpern recommends the adagio (slow) portion of Baroque compositions or his own recordings, like *Spectrum Suite* or *Comfort Zone*.

Although some music therapists believe that any sedate music can help you to relax and calm you, certain songs have a track record. According to a study at the University of South Carolina in Columbia, you may want to stock your CD collection with some Bach, Vivaldi, Debussy, or Mozart. Certain songs by these artists lowered blood pressure, a risk factor for heart disease, says Don Campbell, a music therapist who lectures on the healthful benefits of music, director of the Mozart Effect Resource Center in St. Louis, and author of *The Mozart Effect: Tapping the Power of Music to Heal the Body, Strengthen the Mind, and Unlock the Creative Spirit.*

Use some common scents. Just a whiff of some essential oils can calm you down when you're stressed.

"Either alone or mixed together, lavender, chamomile, peppermint, spearmint, and rosemary may relax you, which could send your blood pressure south," offers Michael Scholes of the Michael Scholes School of Aromatic Studies. So buy products such as candles or a diffuser that will emit the oil scents in your home and office.

Relish a rubdown. Treating yourself to a professional massage every once in awhile will definitely reduce stress, which, in turn, can improve your heart health. But in conjunction with a good diet and exercise, a good circulatory massage may have some added benefits for your heart.

"Massage therapy may help increase a person's circulation. We can help get rid of a lot of the toxic buildup that can occur in the cardiovascular system," says Robert A. Edwards of the Somerset School of Massage Therapy.

High Cholesterol

Playing the Numbers Game

Flip through any number of magazines and you are bound to see it: an ad for cholesterol-lowering drugs. And right behind it are pages of small type detailing the ins, outs, and side effects of these drugs.

It's not that cholesterol-lowering drugs are a bad thing. They have, no doubt, saved many lives and helped those who have cholesterol problems that can only be managed with medication. But for a good number of men, the matter of lowering cholesterol can be done without expensive and side effect–ridden medication. "You only want to be on a drug because you have to. Any drug that is powerful enough to lower cholesterol may sometimes have side effects. If you can prevent it from happening, then that's the way to go," says Gene Spiller, Ph.D., a nutrition researcher, director of the Health Research and Studies Center in Los Altos, California, and co-author of *Nutrition Secrets of the Ancients.*

Take the Cholesterol Test

Cholesterol is a waxy fat made by your liver. Despite its bad press, you need cholesterol to survive. Without it, you couldn't make essential hormones or build cell walls. Your liver makes all the cholesterol you need.

Cholesterol wouldn't be a problem if it wasn't for all the fat you consume. When you eat foods like cheeseburgers and heavily buttered bread, your liver starts churning out more cholesterol—more than you

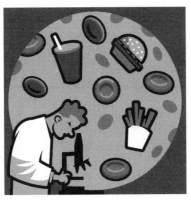

need. Your body can't get rid of this extra cholesterol, so it stores it in your bloodstream. When too much builds up in the bloodstream, it clumps together and attaches to artery walls. That begins to build up and eventually decreases or even blocks off blood flow.

When it comes to measuring your cholesterol, you probably haven't seen so many numbers and letters bantered about since the last time you happened upon *Sesame Street*. Although not that easy to decipher, they do matter to your health, Dr. Spiller says. Here's a quick primer on what they mean.

Total cholesterol: This is the total amount of cholesterol that floats through your bloodstream. A total cholesterol count of 200 milligrams per deciliter of blood or lower is considered healthy, with 160 to 199 milligrams per deciliter being ideal; 200 to 239 is considered borderline high; and anything over 240 is considered high.

HDL cholesterol: HDL is high-density lipoprotein. All you need to understand about HDL is that more is better. This "good" cholesterol removes plaque from your arteries. Men should score more than 45 on an HDL test.

LDL cholesterol: The "L" stands for "low," as in low-density lipoprotein. LDL is the bad guy of cholesterol. It's the LDL that causes hardening of the arteries. Your LDL should be lower than 130. If you already have heart disease, your LDL should be less than 100.

All these numbers and letters mean nothing unless you get tested, Dr. Spiller explains. Make an appointment with your doctor and ask him to test for at least your total and HDL cholesterol levels.

The Envelope, Please

Once you get your numbers, you may find yourself in that upper range. But as Dr.

Spiller says, this is one problem over which you have a certain degree of power. By doing some of the natural, simple things we list below, you may save yourself from high cholesterol, heart disease, and a number of other related problems without medication.

Meddle with meat. Changing the way you prepare food will cut the fat out of your diet without squelching your carnivorous instincts. Try the following, says Laurie Meyer, R.D., a nutritionist in private practice in Milwaukee, some of which can cut up to 50 percent of the fat content.

- Pick your meat wisely. Top round, bottom round, and sirloin tips are leaner meats.
- Cut off exposed fat before you cook the meat.
- Throw meat on the grill so the fat will drip off.
- Brown ground beef, then place it in a dish lined with a double-thickness paper towel. Stick another paper towel on top and blot. The towels will absorb excess fat.
- Choose low-fat roast beef, turkey, or chicken when making a sandwich, rather than high-fat lunchmeats like salami.

Skim down. Look for the words *skim, low-fat,* and *fat-free* when you walk down the dairy aisle, says Meyer. Buy skim and low-fat cheeses, milk, and yogurt. Whole milk gets nearly 50 percent of its calories from fat, and Cheddar cheese gets 74 percent of its calories from fat. Meanwhile, skim milk's fat content is only 6 percent of its total calories.

Make a mono exception. Whenever you would normally use vegetable oil or butter to cook, replace it with olive oil, Meyer suggests. Olive oil contains monounsaturated fatty acids and may raise or maintain your HDL cholesterol and keep LDL from building up and restricting your blood flow. One study in Australia found that a low-fat diet supplemented with olive oil kept HDL levels up while lowering LDL levels. The low-fat diet without the olive oil didn't keep

the HDL from dropping. But remember that fat is still fat and will add to both your cholesterol levels and waistline if not used in moderation.

Snack on nature's candy. Reach for carrot sticks or apples when you feel hungry. By doing so, you'll increase the number of fruits and vegetables in your diet. That will keep your cholesterol down in three ways. First, these foods have no fat. Second, they are full of fiber, which scrubs out the inside of your arteries and gets rid of cholesterol. And third, the fiber fills you up better than a bag of potato chips, which is full of fat, anyway, says Dr. Victor S. Sierpina of the University of Texas Medical Branch.

Bean up. The next time you go to a Mexican eatery, order a bean burrito instead of beef, Meyer suggests. Beans contain soluble fiber, a gumlike substance that sticks to cholesterol then takes it out of your system through the waste process. A number of studies have shown that a diet that includes beans reduces total cholesterol levels anywhere from 10 to 20 percent, says Meyer.

Blend up a soy milkshake. Toss soy milk, fresh fruit, and ice cubes into a blender, and what do you have? A cholesterol-lowering milkshake. Soy foods, such as soy milk and tofu, have been shown to lower cholesterol, says Meyer. In addition to the milkshake, keep a block of tofu in your fridge, she suggests. Come mealtime, cut off a piece, crumble it, and toss it into pasta and stir-fry dishes. Also be on the lookout for tofu burgers in supermarkets and restaurants, Meyer says. Once a week, try a tofu burger instead of reaching for your regular meat fare.

After studying 38 trials, researchers at the University of Kentucky College of Medicine in Lexington found that people with moderately high cholesterol who ate an average of 1½ ounces of soy daily reduced their LDL levels by 12.9 percent, and their total cholesterol 9.3 percent. Soy worked best on the people with the highest cholesterol levels to begin with. The theory behind soy's effect on cholesterol is that it contains phytoestrogens. Phytoestrogens may help take LDL cholesterol from the blood to the liver, where your body gets rid of it.

Garnish with garlic. Garlic does a wonderful job of keeping away annoying people, like vampires and co-workers. It does just as good a job keeping away another annoying and threatening entity—cholesterol. A study of 261 patients with high cholesterol found that 2.8 grams of garlic—about a clove a day—lowered cholesterol levels by an average of 12 percent. Toss the "stinking rose" into your meals, or take 400 milligrams of the dried powder enteric-coated capsule supplements per day to get the garlic without the breath, Dr. Sierpina says.

Stock up the wine rack. A glass of red wine packs a double whammy against cholesterol. First, the alcohol in wine is thought to raise HDL, or the "good," cholesterol in your body. Second, red wine contains antioxidants called polyphenols. These polyphenols keep the LDL cholesterol from sticking to your artery walls and impeding blood flow through your body, says Dr. Joe A. Vinson of the University of Scranton. Remember to keep to just one five-ounce glass of wine per day, or you'll be throwing the benefits out the window.

Have high tea. Tea and red wine don't seem to naturally go together, but when it comes to cholesterol, they do. You can find higher levels of polyphenols in red wine or in tea, Dr. Vinson says. These antioxidants will keep your cholesterol from sticking to your artery walls and making them stiff and narrow. Don't worry about your choice of tea; green, black, and even iced tea have the polyphenols as long as they are brewed, he says. Just don't make it herbal tea, since herb teas don't have enough polyphenols to be effective.

Two Pipes, One Remedy

There is an over-the-counter supplement that can lower your total and low-density lipoprotein (LDL, the "bad") cholesterol. But don't look for it near the vitamins or the promise-packing supplements that work on muscle building and memory enhancement.

Head on over to the laxative section. Yes, that's right. Among the laxatives, you'll find the product that could kick your cholesterol levels down a few notches.

The soluble fiber psyllium is a natural component of some laxatives. But research shows that it does a lot more than keep you regular. In a study of 248 people at the University of Kentucky College of Medicine in Lexington, people who were given a daily psyllium supplement for six months had a more than 8 percent reduction of total cholesterol and an 11 percent reduction in LDL cholesterol. As a soluble fiber, psyllium soaks up the cholesterol floating around your body and takes it out of your system.

The dose used in the study was 5.1 grams of psyllium twice a day—about three rounded teaspoons total. Dr. Victor S. Sierpina of the University of Texas Medical Branch suggests working your way up to that amount by starting with one dose—a rounded teaspoon—a day. After a week or so, gradually move up to two doses. And when you feel comfortable with that, then move on to the third teaspoon. By taking it slowly, you should get used to taking it every day without worrying about its laxative effects.

Caution: Do not take this product if you have difficulty swallowing. If you experience chest pain, vomiting, or difficulty swallowing or breathing after consuming this product, seek immediate medical attention.

Cancer

Cutting Down Your Risk Naturally

Cancer in some form or another used to be thought of as an inevitable consequence of aging. But like many common beliefs, that old-fashioned notion has fallen to the wayside. Now experts believe that most cancers are caused by the world around us—cigarette smoke, exposure to chemicals, poor diet, and lack of exercise. In other words, a good deal of what causes cancer is under your control.

The Best Defense

Nutrition is probably the first and most effective line of defense against cancer. The American Institute of Cancer Research predicts that if the world switched to the right diet, it would prevent anywhere from three to four million new cases of cancer every year. Diet can reduce the risk of developing almost every form of cancer—oral, laryngeal, esophageal, lung, stomach, pancreatic, colon, rectal, prostate, and liver. In addition to diet, other studies have found that supplementing with a common herb and mineral can further reduce your chances.

Don't chew the fat.

A few simple steps can cut a good deal of fat out of your meals, says Melanie R. Polk, R.D., director of nutrition education at the American Institute for Cancer Research in Washington, D.C. She suggests the following:

- Buy skim or low-fat dairy products.
- Keep bottles of flavored vinegars and low-fat salad dressings in the pantry. Use these in order to cut down on oils in marinades for meat and vegetables.
- Spice it up. Add spices and herbs to your cooking—especially vegetables—instead of fats to bring out the flavor.
- Look on the nutrition labels. Select items with less fat, less sodium, and more fiber.

You want to cut down on fat because a number of studies indicate that a high-fat diet may increase the risk of some cancers, especially colon, prostate, and rectal. The American Institute for Cancer Research suggests keeping fats and oils to between 15 and 30 percent of your total calories.

Take this shopping list with you.

The next time you go to the grocery store, fill your cart with produce items such as onions, garlic, carrots, greens, broccoli, cauliflower, and tomatoes. Why these? They are a few of the fruits and vegetables most often linked with reduced cancer rates.

Start your morning with wheat.

Fill your breakfast bowl each morning with a wheat bran cereal like Raisin Bran. Studies have found that wheat bran—the kind found in wheat bran cereal or whole-wheat breads—most consistently offers protection from colon cancer. Fiber from wheat bran increases the bulk of your stool, which ends up diluting cancer-causing agents found there. By increasing the bulk, it speeds up the transit time, meaning that your body gets rid of waste sooner. That leaves a lot less time for those cancer-causing agents to sit in your colon, where they could cause some serious damage. Cereal isn't the only place to get fiber. Substitute whole-wheat breads for white bread; choose brown rice, bulgur, or quinoa instead of white rice; and include at least five servings of fruits and vegetables every day, Polk says.

Toss in some garlic. Learning to cook with garlic and other herbs and spices will improve your culinary skills as well as increase your protection from cancer, Polk explains. Invest in a garlic press, a tool that crushes garlic into bits, and throw mashed cloves into stir-fry and pasta meals, she suggests. Use it as an added flavor to vegetable dishes, too.

Prostate Protection

Prostate cancer rates have doubled in the past two decades, and that's possibly a good thing. Why? It's likely that the actual incidence of prostate cancer hasn't risen. It's the number of men and their doctors paying attention to prostate cancer that has increased, so more cases are diagnosed than ever before. Early detection and annual screenings after age 50 are the best defense against prostate cancer.

You also have the power to lower your odds of developing the second leading cause of death among American men. The foods you eat and the supplements you take play a role in the health of your prostate, says Warren Heston, Ph.D., director of the George M. O'Brien Urology Research Center at the Memorial Sloan-Kettering Cancer Center in New York City.

Say tomato. Go heavy on the sauce the next time you order a pizza. A few years ago, a study came out proclaiming the tomato as the superpower of the prostate. The Harvard study of more than 48,000 men found that men who ate at least 10 servings of tomato-based foods a week reduced their risks of prostate cancer by 45 percent. The foods with the highest reduction in prostate cancer risk were tomato sauce, tomatoes, and pizza. The researchers have attributed this finding to the amount of lycopene that is found in tomatoes. Lycopene is a carotenoid that gives tomatoes their red color.

Don't just load up the pantry with tomato paste, warns Dr. Heston. It may be something else in the tomatoes that protects the prostate. To be truly safe, mix a nice dose of tomato products into a diet already filled with a variety of fruits and vegetables, he says.

Take vitamin E. Take at least 75 international units of vitamin E a day, Dr. Heston suggests. Vitamin E supplements have been recommended for their positive effects on the heart, but another study has found that the antioxidant may also protect your prostate. A study of more than 29,000 men in Finland found that those who took 50 milligrams of vitamin E—about 75 international units—a day had a 32 percent lower incidence of prostate cancer than those who did not take the supplement had. The death rate from the disease was 41 percent lower among the men who took vitamin E as well. "This level of vitamin E supplement has a potential benefit," Dr. Heston says.

Keep your folate up. Get your Daily Value of 400 micrograms of folate. You can easily get 400 micrograms of folic acid—the supplement form of folate—by taking a multivitamin with that amount, Dr. Heston says. You can also get folate from green leafy vegetables like spinach and turnip greens; beans, especially lentils, kidney beans, lima beans, and pinto beans; asparagus; wheat germ; chicken liver; and fortified breakfast cereals. Why folate? Although more research is needed, getting enough folate may turn out to be a key in preventing prostate cancer, Dr. Heston says.

In your prostate swims a protein called folate hydrolase. There's more of this folate hydrolase in your prostate than in any other area of your body, says Dr. Heston. These folate hydrolase proteins prevent the B vitamin folate from staying inside the prostate cells. Eventually, because the folate leaks out of them, these prostate cells develop a folate deficiency, Dr. Heston says. When the cells lack the folate, it makes it easier for cancer-causing agents to take hold and develop. Dr. Heston and his researchers believe that this folate deficiency may be a major factor in the development of prostate cancer.

Back Pain

Getting Your Back into Shape

Your back is home to about 200 muscles and 33 bones—that's about 233 ways for something to go wrong. And a lot does go wrong. About 90 percent of Americans will experience at least one back pain incident in their lifetimes.

Lying perfectly still for hours and even days may be what you feel like doing during a back pain episode, but it's not the best thing you can do, says Dennis C. Turk, Ph.D., John and Emma Bonica professor of anesthesiology and pain research at the University of Washington School of Medicine in Seattle. Long-term inactivity is possibly one of the worst ways to treat back pain. A few days on your back actually weakens back muscles. Instead of taking it lying down, be open to some of these New Age and age-old natural remedies that your doctor might not be aware of.

Become a Dough Boy

If you want to prevent back problems, treat your back like a pizza chef treats his pizza dough. Knead it a bit, stretch it a bit, pull on it a bit, and apply direct but gentle pressure. To do this, mix up a little massage, acupressure, and even some yoga. Here's how.

Roll around. If your game isn't up to par lately, you can still put all your tennis and golf balls to good use. Grab a tennis ball (for beginners) or a golf ball (for advanced folks) to give yourself a quick and easy back massage. Either sitting in a chair or lying down, take the ball and place it behind your lower back or wherever you feel pain. Then roll around and move your back so that the ball rubs into your back muscles. "It will cause some relief," says Robert A. Edwards of the Somerset School of Massage Therapy. If at any time you feel pain, either let up on the ball or stop, he adds. Edwards suggests rolling around for two to three minutes twice a day.

Bend your back muscles. Stretching your back muscles helps you create a greater range of movement. It also enhances the elasticity of your muscles and spinal joints, says the Acupressure Institute's Dr. Michael Reed Gach, author of *The Bum Back Book*. Here's a basic stretch and a good starting point: Stand with your hands behind your lower back for support and your knees slightly bent. Slowly bend backward, far enough to get a gentle stretch. Exhale as you bend. Then, come back up very slowly, keeping your knees bent, while you inhale. Do this exercise daily, stretching the spine several times. If this gentle exercise aggravates your back pain, stop it and consult a doctor or physical therapist, advises Dr. Gach.

Stretch back your back. This acupressure move stimulates several key trigger points in your upper back and loosens the knots that tend to cause pain, Dr. Gach says: Interlace your hands with your palms facing each other behind your back near your buttocks. As you inhale deeply, stretch your arms away from your back, pressing your shoulder blades together. Hold for a few seconds. Repeat this exercise three more times, and do it twice a day, says Dr. Gach.

Make some heat. Using either your palms or the backs of your hands, rub your lower back until you generate heat. "The friction will warm the area and increase circulation," Dr. Gach says. By rubbing the entire lower-back area, you inevitably stimulate many of the acupressure points located there, Dr. Gach adds. This will activate those points and will ease some of your pain.

Strike a pose. Several yoga poses can help relieve back pain while also strengthening your back to prevent further problems. "Many of the poses in yoga are especially beneficial for spinal health. Some are the same exercises suggested by back-care specialists and physical therapists," says yoga instructor Mara Carrico. The classic knee-to-chest pose helps relieve common lower-back discomfort, she adds. Lie on your back with your arms at your sides. Place a folded towel under your head to keep your neck and head in line with your spine. Bring your right knee up to your chest. Place your clasped hands underneath your right knee. Relax your right foot. Straighten your left leg on the floor as you flex your left foot. Keep your head centered and relax your shoulders. Hold this pose for 20 to 60 seconds, and then do the same exercise with the left leg. Try to do at least two sets every day, Carrico suggests.

Make like a snake. The cobra pose is a common hatha yoga posture that helps strengthen the spine and back, Carrico says. Lying on your stomach, bend your elbows and place your hands underneath your shoulders. Keep your legs hip-distance apart. Tighten your buttocks. As you inhale, straighten your arms to raise your chest up, and look forward while keeping your hips and the rest of your lower body on the floor. Then exhale. Don't let your shoulders tense toward your ears, she cautions. If you need to, keep your elbows slightly bent, Carrico suggests. Hold this position for a few breaths (10 to 20 seconds). When you are ready to release, exhale. Do this two or three times every day, Carrico suggests.

Back Pain: You Can Stick It

In the clenches of a back pain attack, sticking a bunch of needles all over your body may not sound like a viable solution. But it just might be what you're looking for. Back pain sends many people to the acupuncturist. "I have treated many patients for back pain *after* their back surgery. It would have been beneficial to spare them the surgery since they still had pain afterward," says Dr. Victor S. Sierpina of the University of Texas Medical Branch.

Acupuncture has made its name in the United States as a treatment for back pain and other chronic conditions. In one study, 50 people with chronic lower-back pain were separated into two groups. One group received acupuncture treatment right away, while the other group had to wait awhile. Eighty-three percent of the group treated immediately reported that their pain was cut in half. While the other group waited, only about 33 percent reported feeling better, and 25 percent reported that their pain got worse. Once the second group received acupuncture, 75 percent of them reported that their pain was alleviated.

To find a qualified acupuncturist, look for certification by the National Commission for the Certification of Acupuncture and Oriental Medicine or an M.D. with at least 200 hours of training.

Getting Back in the Saddle

Traditionally, the prescription to fix back pain consisted of taking it easy, propping your legs up, and reaching for some acetaminophen and the television remote control. You felt pretty powerless. But you can take action to speed up your healing time, and for the most part, you don't have to get out of your chair to do it.

Work on your feet. According to reflexology, the art of improving your health by manipulating pressure points in your feet, the midway point down the inner sides of your foot represents the spine and back area. By pressing on that special point, you can relieve some of your back pain. How do you find this precise spot? Instead of memorizing the special reflexology chart, just give yourself a foot rub down those inner sides when you have back pain, Edwards says. "If you find a point that is extremely tender, then you know you have it," he says. Once you find that point, gradually increase the amount of pressure.

Go hot and cold. Its technical name is hydrotherapy, but all it means is using water to soothe your sore back. Alternate hot and cold packs for about 15 minutes on your back when it hurts, Edwards says. Get extra relief by soaking in a warm bath then applying a cold compress. "A warm bath is relaxing and soothing," he adds, while the cold compress helps minimize pain.

Oil yourself up. The essential oils of birch, wintergreen, and peppermint can help calm back pain, says Michael Scholes of the Michael Scholes School of Aromatic Studies. But if you're going to use them, you must dilute essential oils in a carrier base oil such as jojoba, baby, or castor oil (10 to 12 drops of essential oil per ounce of carrier oil). Then have someone massage them into your back to help alleviate pain, according to Scholes.

You can also put a few drops of peppermint on a compress and place it against the sore area of your back. Peppermint gets the circulation moving and the blood flowing to the injured area, he explains.

Reach for your knees. An acupressure point located in the center of the crease in

Taking a Crack at Chiropractic

The way chiropractors see it, nobody knows more about your back than they do. The basis of their entire practice lies in the spine. According to chiropractic medicine, joints and vertebrae get knocked out of line, or lock in one position, and cause different conditions, including back pain.

Using his hands, the chiropractor pushes or adjusts the problem back into place or into a normal movement. "It is a gentle process. The motion is very easy and not deep," says Jerome F. McAndrews, D.C., a spokesperson for the American Chiropractic Association in Arlington, Virginia. Depending on the injury, it may take one session or it may take several, he says.

That said, a little prevention can minimize your need to see a chiropractor. To keep your joints, vertebrae, and

the back of the knee can relieve back pain. Using your fingers, find the center of the crease. Apply firm pressure with your fingers at different angles, until you feel a rather sharp sensation.

"This usually takes some gentle poking around," Dr. Gach says. When you feel the sensation, you have the point. Hold that point for about two minutes, slowly inhaling and exhaling. After doing one side, switch to the other, Dr. Gach says. For best results, do both knees three times a day.

Press pain away. Another acupressure point for back pain is located on the outside of your ankle between the ankle bone and your heel, Dr. Gach says.

Place your thumb on the outside of your right ankle, and place your index finger on the inside of your ankle, as if you were pinching your ankle. Slide your thumb and press it into the soft tissue in the back of your heel bone.

back muscles in proper alignment, Dr. McAndrews recommends the following.

Don't sit for long periods of time. Even if you have a desk job, get up and take a walk every hour or so, Dr. McAndrews says. This keeps the muscles in your lower back and legs from shortening, which can cause back pain, he says.

Lift with your legs, not your back. And never lift with your head turned, he warns. By turning your head while lifting, you contort your spine in more than one way at a time, which contributes to back pain.

Ease up on the support. If you wear a support belt at work, take it off or loosen it when you aren't lifting. "The muscles will become dependent on the belt. Don't let those muscles weaken," he says.

Hold the pressure for at least two minutes. Shake out the ankle before doing the same thing to your left side. Keep your breathing deep and slow during the exercise. Repeat this exercise three times a day for best results, suggests Dr. Gach.

Stick your finger in your ear. There is an acupressure point inside the top of your ear—called the neurogate point—that can control back pain, says certified acupuncturist Dr. David Nickel.

The neurogate point is located in the middle of the upper part of the ear, just above the main ear opening. Press the point firmly for five seconds, then let go for five seconds, Dr. Nickel recommends. Stick with the five-second intervals for one full minute. Exhale through your mouth as you apply the pressure, and inhale through your nose as you ease off the pressure point. If you can't find the exact point, press all over your ear until you hit a tender spot, Dr. Nickel suggests. Repeat the exercises two or three times a day or as needed for relief of pain, he says.

Try a little tenseness. Back pain usually doesn't strike out of the blue. You've probably been building up that painful feeling over days or weeks of muscle tension that climaxes into a spasm or a really sore back. "Many times, we don't even know we're tense until it is too late and our back starts to spasm. So teach yourself what tension feels like," says Dr. Turk. Sitting in a chair or wherever you feel comfortable, intentionally tense up your back muscles.

"Think about what it feels like to be tight and tense. Then release and think about what it feels like to be loose," he suggests. Every once in awhile, make a spot check of your back muscles. Do they feel tense or loose? If they are tense, use relaxation or stretching exercises to reduce the tension and cut the pain off at the pass, Dr. Turk says.

Relax your mind and back. During your next back pain attack, try the following exercise: Sit in a chair and focus on your breathing. Slowly inhale, hold the breath for a second, then exhale as if you are blowing on a candle flame but don't want to blow it out. As you do this, picture yourself sinking into the chair. Think about feeling warmth and heaviness near your back.

"The warmth helps relieve pain and tension," Dr. Turk says. Do this for two to five minutes a few times a day, he suggests. "Whenever you feel tense or stressed or your pain increases, take a short break, even one to two minutes, at work, at home, wherever. This is a portable approach that can be done anywhere, as needed," he explains. This should help relieve some of the pain as well as relax your entire body and mind, Dr. Turk adds.

Sexual Concerns

Putting Problems to Bed

"Trouble in paradise."

That's how a psychologist once described sex problems in marriage, although it's a phrase that could easily refer to any sex problem. After all, if there's nothing quite so emotionally and physically satisfying as making love, there's nothing quite so emotionally and physically frustrating as not being able to make love successfully. "Paradise lost" might be a better way to put it.

It is no wonder, then, that medical science has spent millions of dollars in research and development, feverishly developing a host of high-tech remedies for every sexual problem under the covers—from pumps and pills to injections that will give you instant erections, first time, every time, no questions asked.

Overlooked in all the hullabaloo about these quick fixes is the fact that there are plenty of things you can do to deal with sex problems without using drugs or machines. Here's an overview of some of the most common sexual problems affecting men today, and some of the natural remedies you can use to address them.

Impotence

Erectile dysfunction, as doctors now prefer to call it, affects an estimated 18 million American men. The more important statistic is this one: 80 to 90 percent of chronic potency problems have a physical basis, usually having something to do with the heart or circulatory system. "Your penis is hooked up to same blood vessels every-

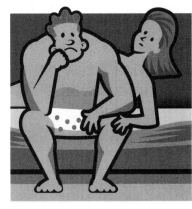

thing else is, so whatever affects your blood supply can affect your penis, too," says Joseph Oesterling, M.D., director of the Midwest Prostate Institute in Saginaw, Michigan.

The message is clear: Whatever you can do to keep your heart happily pumping is going to help keep your penis happily rising. Here are some specific suggestions.

Be heart-smart. "Follow the basic building blocks of good health," says urologist Kenneth Goldberg, M.D., founder and director of the Male Health Institute in Irving, Texas. That means keeping your cardiovascular system in good shape by getting 30 minutes of regular aerobic exercise every day, eating a low-fat diet, and not smoking.

Gobble some vitamins. Taking the antioxidant vitamins C and E and beta-carotene (which the body turns into vitamin A) will also help promote good cardiovascular health, Dr. Goldberg says. Look for a multivitamin, or take supplements that will give you 1,000 milligrams a day of vitamin C, 400 international units of vitamin E, and 25,000 international units of beta-carotene, he says.

If you are considering taking vitamin E in amounts above 200 international units, discuss this with your doctor first. One study using low-dose vitamin E supplements showed an increased risk of hemorrhagic stroke.

Go get ginkgo. One of the best-known herbal remedies for improving blood circulation to the brain is ginkgo biloba. But it also seems to boost blood flow into the penis, thus aiding iffy erections, according to retired botanist Dr. James A. Duke. In one study, physicians obtained good results with 60 to 240 milligrams daily of a standardized ginkgo extract. In that study, 78 men with impotence as a result of clogged penile arteries reported significant improvement without side effects after remaining on this herbal extract for nine months.

Don't expect immediate results with ginkgo, warns Dr. Duke. The best way to use this herb is to buy a standardized extract of capsules. Look for standardized gingko with 24 percent flavonoid glycosides and 6 percent gingkolides at a health food store or drugstore, he says. He recommends taking 60 to 240 milligrams of standardized ginkgo extract a day, but don't go any higher than that, he cautions. Taking too much concentrated gingko extract can cause dermatitis, diarrhea, and vomiting. This herb may increase the action of pharmaceutical monoamine oxidase (MAO) inhibitors, such as Nardil.

Intimacy and Stress

Everything we've just told you about how erections depend on good cardiovascular health is true, but that's not the whole story. Any man who has a problem getting it up and doesn't react emotionally to that experience can be sure that he has discovered the source of his trouble: He's dead.

Along with physical problems, the other main factor is lack of desire. "That accounts for more than half my practice, and the same is probably true for other sex therapists," says Shirley Zussman, Ed.D., a certified sex and marital therapist in private practice in New York City.

What accounts for this epidemic of the sexual blahs? Boredom, depression, marital tension, and stress are the most frequent reasons, says Dr. Zussman. The question is what do you do about it? Here are some suggestions for keeping this Murderer's Row of modern problems from messing up your love life.

Talk it out. You don't necessarily have to go into therapy to get help for mild depression, Dr. Zussman says, but you should do something about it. The depressed partner needs to find someone—the other partner, a friend, a family member, a religious leader—to talk to. "Don't just let it go on," she says, "be-cause depression isn't an incurable state, and we shouldn't have to live with it."

Serious depression, Dr. Zussman adds, should be addressed professionally. Be aware, however, that many antidepressant drugs can actually lower your sex drive, not raise it.

Shake it up. If you've fallen into a sexual rut, find a new groove, Dr. Zussman says. "Tell her, 'Look, we've been having some great sex, but let's see if there is something different we can do. Let's change the time, place, and pace of it.'"

Do the spoon. Touching another human can release hormones that promote feelings of intimacy and social connection. One way to take advantage of that physiological truth is to practice "the nurturing meditation," says Charles Muir, a longtime teacher of Tantra, director of the Source School of Tantra Yoga in Paia, Hawaii, and co-author of *Tantra: The Art of Conscious Loving.*

Lie on your side with your partner spoon-fashion. (Tantric texts recommend the left side, Muir says, to enhance energy flow.) The partner on the inside—the man or the woman, whoever needs nurturing most—is enveloped in the arms of the partner on the outside. Muir recommends assuming this position at the beginning and at the end of each day.

The nurturing meditation can proceed to sex, Muir says, but it doesn't have to. "The purpose of the nurturing position is to create balance and harmony between the two partners," he says.

Have a heart. Another method that Muir recommends for promoting intimacy is the "hands on heart" meditation. The woman places one hand flat in the center of the man's chest and massages him there with a gentle circular motion. She should look into his eyes while doing so. Her other hand can be placed on his back, or she can use it to cup his testicles. "A lot of energy is stuffed in men's heart center," Muir says. "Men have learned how to be hard on the outside, but they're often kind of hollow on the inside because they don't know how to feel loved."

Draw your relationship.
Sometimes words can hinder rather than help communication between partners, because they can create misunderstandings or because we don't realize ourselves what's really going on in our hearts, says Linda Gantt, Ph.D., director of art therapy at the Trauma Recovery Institute in Morgantown, West Virginia, and past president of the American Art Therapy Association, which is headquartered in Mundelein, Illinois. Drawing a picture of our relationship can help circumvent those mental blocks to reveal hidden truths.

Each partner should sit down in the same room and try drawing his experience of sex: before, during, and after. Don't look at each other's drawings until you're both finished, Dr. Gantt says. "That way each person gets his own say, which is especially important if one partner tends to verbally dominate the relationship."

When you're both finished, it's time for show and tell. Look at each other's drawings, discuss them, and try to analyze what you think they mean, paying attention to the colors, shapes, themes, and moods that emerge. Also, notice how the drawings differ and how they're similar.

The goal of this exercise is mutual understanding and insight, Dr. Gantt says. Your drawings may provide an emotional road map, of sorts, that will help you improve your relationship. Once you're done, make a drawing together.

Pray for strength. Your relationship will be strengthened if you and your partner pray together, suggests Michael J. McManus, president of Marriage Savers, an organization in Bethesda, Maryland, that works with churches to reduce the incidence of divorce, who writes a syndicated column entitled "Ethics and Religion." Praying regularly for solutions to the

In Pursuit of Sexual Alchemy

The search for a genuine aphrodisiac has been a quest of humankind for thousands of years, causing everything from dried rhinoceros horn to dried beetles to be packaged and sold as the fountain of sexual youth. The results so far have not lived up to the legends, although a host of herbs are still reputed to have aphrodisiac effects.

By far the most promising contender is a derivative of the bark of the African yohimbe tree, says retired botanist Dr. James A. Duke. In its natural form, yohimbe has some serious side effects, including anxiety, increased heart rate, elevated blood pressure, hallucinations, and headache. But a safer, standardized version is available by prescription. Some studies have shown that it helps restore erections for some men with erection problems, which is not the same as saying it stimulates desire in men who don't have such problems. Even there, the evidence is mixed, and researchers suspect that the herb's effects may be more psychological than physiological.

The same might be said of those aphrodisiac concoc-

toughest problems will lead to solutions and a reduction in overall stress, McManus says. Since the book of Proverbs is filled with practical advice in 31 chapters, he recommends reading a chapter together each morning. After reflecting on it, each partner can pray for the other to make it peacefully and successfully through the day. "What this does is build intimacy at a spiritual level," McManus says, "and that can only help with other forms of intimacy."

The Prostate Prescription

Lots of middle-aged men spend more time thinking about their prostate glands than

tions that fill the shelves of health food stores these days. Such products as "Cobra" and "Deepak's Libidoplex" feature a wide range of herbs that have been credited traditionally, not scientifically, with aphrodisiac qualities. A typical mixture might contain some combination of yohimbe, ginger, ginseng, nettle, alfalfa, muira puama, and saw palmetto, among other things.

Do they work? It's hard to say, according to Dr. Duke. The herbs involved have earned their reputations through folklore, not science, he says. But the folks who invented the folklore didn't necessarily throw their individual remedies into a big aphrodisiac stew. "Nobody knows whether these mixtures are canceling each other out through antagonisms or augmenting each other through synergisms," he says.

Still, these love potions may well work on the same principle that aphrodisiacs through the ages have generally worked: by the placebo effect. "If people believe they'll do the trick, they probably will," says Dr. Duke.

they want to, mainly because the darned things cause so many of them to have to keep getting up in the middle of the night to urinate.

The problem is benign prostatic hyperplasia, or BPH. What that means is that the prostate swells, but it's a benign condition—that is, it doesn't lead to cancer, Dr. Oesterling explains. BPH is a remarkably common condition: At least half of men older than 50 have it. By the time we hit our seventies, the numbers go up to 80 percent.

As with impotence, there are plenty of heavy-duty drugs that you can take to deal with BPH, and surgery is an option. But there's a kinder, gentler way to handle the problem: saw palmetto.

The saw palmetto berry is an herb that's native to the United States. It was first used hundreds of years ago by the Seminole Indians, who considered it a potent aphrodisiac. Now, however, it has become widely accepted as a treatment for BPH, and for good reason: It works. "I'd bet my prostate on it," says Dr. Duke. "I can count a good number of scientific studies done over the past decade that indicate that saw palmetto can help relieve symptoms in men with BPH."

If you have mild symptoms of swollen prostate—if you get up several times a night to urinate, for example, or if you feel you have to run to the rest room when the urge hits—here are some guidelines for using the saw palmetto solution.

Check with your doctor first. Saw palmetto should be taken under a doctor's guidance, after receiving a definite diagnosis of BPH, cautions Andrew Weil, M.D., director of the Program in Integrative Medicine at the University of Arizona College of Medicine in Tucson. If your doctor resists the idea of using herbal remedies, be politely persistent, Dr. Weil says. If he still refuses, "you may need to seek out a doctor with a more open mind or more knowledge of herbal medicine."

Go the standard route. The best way to take saw palmetto is to use a standardized oil-based extract, says Varro E. Tyler, Ph.D., distinguished professor emeritus of pharmacognosy and dean emeritus of Purdue University School of Pharmacy and Pharmacal Sciences in West Lafayette, Indiana. Look for brands that say they're standardized to 85 to 95 percent fatty acids and sterols, and take 320 milligrams a day.

As with most herbal remedies, be patient: It can take several weeks of treatment for BPH symptoms to improve.

Headache

Tackling Headaches Head-On

Headaches evoke such sympathetic responses because almost everyone gets them at some time. In one year alone, more than nine million Americans of all ages went to doctors because of headaches. Headaches rank as the number one reason that Americans reach for over-the-counter painkillers. Researchers estimate that 60 percent of all U.S. adults took painkillers for headaches during a six-month period.

All that pill popping may not be the best thing for your aching head. Over-the-counter analgesics have been linked with making headaches worse and with causing rebound headaches after the medication wears off. There are other less invasive ways of trying to stop the drumbeat in your head. In the midst of your next headache, give some of the following natural remedies a try.

Soothe sinus headaches. Trace your eyebrows to massage away sinus and headache pain, says Robert A. Edwards of the Somerset School of Massage Therapy. Using your fingers, massage in a circular motion starting between your eyebrows, above your nose. Slowly move the massaging motion out toward the sides of your head. Massage right below your eyebrows. Do this several times on each eyebrow, Edwards suggests.

Give it a pinch. Right at the top of your earlobe, where the fleshy part of your ear meets the harder cartilage, hides the headache ear point for acupressure. Put your forefinger on this point and your thumb behind it and squeeze. For best results, pinch hard enough to experience a "good" hurt—a hot stinging sensation. Squeeze the point firmly for five seconds, then let up for five seconds, says certified acupuncturist Dr. David Nickel. Keep with the five-second intervals for a full minute. Exhale through your mouth as you apply the pressure, and inhale through your nose as you ease off the pressure point. If you can't find the exact point, press all over your ear until you hit a tender spot, Dr. Nickel recommends.

Compress your brain. During a headache, you may feel like grabbing your head and squeezing out the pain. That just might help. Pressing against your skull activates several acupressure points that can alleviate headaches. Place your palms on the sides of your skull, says Dr. Michael Reed Gach of the Acupressure Institute. Then gently press inward toward the center of your head. Press in gradually for several seconds and breathe deeply, he recommends. Keep doing this all around your skull, especially in areas where you feel the most pain.

Point and push. One finger-width above the middle of your eyebrows lies another headache acupressure point, Dr. Gach says. Unlike the firm direct pressure you apply on many acupressure points, be gentle with this one, he advises. Place the tips of your fingers lightly on the point and cover your eyes with your palms. Use a gentle touch instead of pressure, and relax your neck, allowing your head to slump forward. "As you breathe deeply, imagine that you are emptying your mind and letting yourself relax," Dr. Gach says. Hold the point for a minute or two.

Grab a handful. This acupressure point is famous for headache relief. You'll find it in the webbing between the thumb and the index finger, at the highest spot of the muscle that protrudes when the thumb and index finger are brought together. Press that point firmly with your thumb on the top of your hand and your finger underneath. Direct the pressure underneath the bone that attaches to your index finger, Dr. Gach says. "This may hurt a bit, but it indicates that you are on the right point," he says. Hold the point for a minute or two on each hand.

Get toe-tal relief. In reflexology, the tip of each toe activates pain control in your head, Edwards says. Massage and press the tip of each toe during a headache encounter, he suggests. These points should relieve some of the pain and may be able to prevent future headaches.

Bark up a different tree. The willow bark herb is the father of modern aspirin. Commission E, a group of experts that studies herbs for the German government, endorses willow as an effective headache pain reliever. It acts as an analgesic, antipyretic (fever reducer), and anti-inflammatory. Take willow as a tea during the occasional headache, not as a preventive measure, says Dr. Victor S. Sierpina of the University of Texas Medical Branch. To prepare, steep 1 to 1½ teaspoons of dried willow bark in a cup of boiling water for 15 minutes. If you are allergic or sensitive to aspirin, you shouldn't take aspirin-like herbs, either. And you should be aware that if aspirin upsets your stomach, willow bark may do the same. Also, never give either aspirin or its natural herbal alternatives to children who have headaches, as there is a chance that they might develop Reye's syndrome, a potentially fatal condition that damages the liver and brain.

Scent your scalp. When you feel a headache coming on, reach for some lavender and marjoram essential oils, advises Michael Scholes of the Michael Scholes School of Aromatic Studies. Mix together 5 to 6 drops of each

Mitigating Migraines

The following two supplements may help prevent migraine attacks.

Feverfew. This herb from the dandelion and marigold family has been used to prevent and treat migraines and headaches.

If you have migraines, take it as a preventive measure, says Dr. Victor S. Sierpina of the University of Texas Medical Branch. Take two or three 60-milligram capsules of the fresh powdered leaves a day, or two 25-milligram capsules of the freeze-dried leaf daily, he recommends.

Vitamin B$_2$. A heavy dose of a common B vitamin may keep migraines from coming. A study by the Belgium Migraine Society found that taking 400 milligrams of vitamin B$_2$, also known as riboflavin, prevented migraines. Those who took the B$_2$ in the study reported one-third fewer migraines than the placebo group. Although riboflavin is very safe and effective, you'd have to take an entire bottle to get 400 milligrams over-the-counter. Don't do that; get a doctor's prescription to get 400 milligrams, says Marc Lenaerts, M.D., the study co-author and a neurology resident at the University of Oklahoma in Oklahoma City.

essential oil in an ounce of carrier oil such as jojoba, canola, or even a light body lotion. Massage it into your scalp. The two oils may help offset your headache. The scents may help you relax and break the tension that could be exacerbating your headache. Because some essential oils can irritate people with sensitive skin, it is best to talk to a professional aromatherapist to find which oils are right for you.

Seek out the classics. Mozart's music may be able to send your headache away, says Don Campbell of the Mozart Effect Resource

Center. Campbell tells the story of a woman with severe headaches who was desperate for relief. At the instruction of a music therapist, she began listening to Mozart's Symphony no. 39 in E-flat and Symphony no. 12 in A Major. After she listened to the music for awhile, her headaches went away, he says. "For stress-related headaches, music is a great complementary therapy, when used as an adjunct to your traditional headache remedies." Experiment to find music that is soothing to you. The music should be soft, quiet, and melodious, he adds.

Turn down the bass. Maybe you're one of those guys who loves to crank up the bass on your stereo system. If you are, that's not helping your headache at all. "A strong pounding beat will exaggerate and amplify a headache because it will literally cause your heart to pump harder, thereby pumping more blood into the brain, making your headache worse," says Dr. Steven Halpern of Inner Peace Music. Lay off the bass and listen to some softer, slower soothing music, he advises.

Mystery of the Brain Freeze

You've been waiting for it all day. It's hot, and you're hot, as you waltz up to the counter and ask the clerk for a cherry slushie. You slurp through the straw, and as your tastebuds dance with pleasure—bang!—a stabbing pain hits you behind the eye. Brain freeze. Another example of how life's pleasure and pain are so inexplicably linked.

Brain freeze usually occurs a few seconds after you eat or drink something very cold, and it lasts for 30 to 60 seconds. Studies have pinpointed the problem to the soft palate, the roof of your mouth toward your throat, says Joseph Hulihan, M.D., assistant professor of neurology and director of the Headache Center at the Temple University Health Sciences Center in Philadelphia. "The body reads the cold stimulation as pain," Dr. Hulihan says. Studies have also found that people who have migraines experience brain freeze more than others, he added.

A brain freeze or an ice cream headache is what experts call a referred pain. Referred pain is when something

Get Tough on Tension

It doesn't take much to set a tension headache into motion: anxiety, stress, sitting too long in the same position, injuries, eating too much—the list goes on. One or a combination of these events tightens the muscles in your scalp, face, neck, or shoulders. All that tension eventually culminates in one pounding headache that feels like someone is tightening a strap around your head. In a study of more than 13,000 people, 38 percent reported that they had had a tension headache in the past year, and half of those people said that it kept them from functioning properly.

Tension headaches give you warning signals—a stiff neck, tight shoulders. If you heed these signals, you may be able to keep yourself from suffering. These tension-reducing tips can prevent you from getting a tension headache, and they can be used during one as well.

Get back into mint condition. Some headaches really start in your upper back, shoulders, and neck. Because of stress, bad posture, or injury, your back and neck muscles tense and end up triggering a headache. When you have a headache that feels like it sprouted from your neck, take a drop or two of peppermint oil, mix it into another body oil or lotion, and massage it into your shoulders and neck, Scholes says. Peppermint oil may help defuse your tension.

happens in one part of your body, but you feel the pain in another.

In the case of an ice cream headache, the extreme cold hits nerve endings in your soft palate. The soft palate and your head share nerve pathways, so the pain response travels to your head instead of your mouth, Dr. Hulihan says.

Although not dangerous, ice cream headaches sure take the fun out of ice cream. So Dr. Hulihan has a few suggestions to avoid this dilemma.

Let the ice cream or slushie melt a bit. That way it won't be as cold when it hits your mouth.

Don't let the cold stuff hit your soft palate. When you're eating or drinking something cold, keep it around your tongue.

Don't eat slushies with a straw. When you suck in the slushy stuff, the straw shoots it right at your soft palate. You're just aiming for a brain freeze. Go for it with a spoon.

For a headache located right in your temples, take a drop or two of peppermint oil, dilute it in a base oil or lotion, and rub it into your temples, Scholes says. People who have sensitive skin should do a small skin patch test first and then proceed, as directed above, if there is no adverse reaction, says Scholes.

Stretch your neck. Defuse a tension headache by doing some stretches a few times a day, Edwards says. This will keep tension from building up into a king-size headache. For the first exercise, sit in a chair and look forward. Stretch your right arm over your head, place your right hand over your left ear, and pull your head down toward your right shoulder. Hold for about 10 seconds. Then place your left hand over your right ear and

pull down. Repeat five times on each side, Edwards recommends.

After doing the neck stretch, try a variation on head rolls, Edwards says. Focus on a spot right in front of you. Then drop your head forward and roll it over to your right shoulder. "Look up over your shoulder as if you were trying to read the clock on the wall behind you," Edwards says. Roll your head forward again toward the middle, and then roll it over to your left side and look behind your left shoulder.

Get five in one. Five acupressure points for headaches sit at the base of your skull where the back of your neck meets your head. You can make contact with all of them by massaging that hollowed-out area along the base of your skull. Keep your head tilted slightly backward while your fingers press forward at the base of the head, Dr. Gach says. Hold for about two minutes, or until you feel a pulsation, which indicates that energy is flowing to the area, Dr. Gach says.

Practice perfect posture. Bad posture puts a lot of pressure on your back and internal organs. After awhile, all that tension can lead to a headache.

"Men's upper-body muscle mass often leads to tight shoulders and, in turn, neck tension," says yoga instructor Mara Carrico. To correct your improper posture, try the following yoga exercise, called the pose of balance. Stand with your feet hip-width apart, toes pointed forward, and arms at your sides. Make sure your shoulders are relaxed and your chin is parallel to the floor.

Distribute your body weight evenly between your toes and your heels. Keep your kneecaps relaxed. Draw in your abdominal muscles. Drop your shoulders away from your ears, lower your chin a bit, and lengthen the back of your neck. Hold for 30 to 60 seconds, Carrico suggests.

Allergies and Asthma

Breathing in a Polluted and Pollinated World

For the most part, allergies and asthma are nothing more than a mistake made by your immune system. When you breathe in an offending particle, your immune system mistakes the particle for an infectious agent and goes into attack mode, releasing a chemical called histamine that causes your eyes to water, your nose to stuff up, or your airways to constrict. Your role in this war is to send your immune system into retreat. Here are all-natural nondrug methods to do that.

Set up a sting. The stinging nettle herb is nature's antihistamine drug. "There are a number of anecdotal reports about stinging nettle and allergies," says Dr. Victor S. Sierpina of the University of Texas Medical Branch. The nettle root and leaves have antihistamine properties that limit the release of histamine and free up your breathing pathways. Take the stinging nettle herb when your allergies start or when you feel an asthma attack coming on, he recommends. Put two teaspoons of the dried herb in a cup of boiling water and steep for 10 to 15 minutes. Drink one cup of the tea once every four hours until your symptoms clear up, Dr. Sierpina says.

Drown symptoms in vitamin C. High levels of vitamin C help keep histamine in check and also make histamine break down faster once it is released. Doses of about 3,000 milligrams of vitamin C help

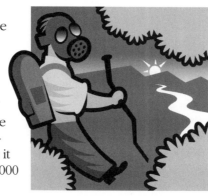

reduce the symptoms of asthma and allergies, especially seasonal allergies, says clinical nutritionist Dr. Shari Lieberman. Spread the dosages throughout the day by taking about 1,000 milligrams with each meal. When your allergies or asthma problems subside, you can cut down to 500 to 1,000 milligrams of vitamin C a day for maintenance, or you may stay on the higher 3,000-milligram dose, she says. Be aware that excessive vitamin C may cause diarrhea in some people.

Press under your collarbone. To relieve the congestion and breathing problems associated with asthma, feel for your collarbone. Place your fingertips in the hollows directly below the protrusions on either side of the collarbone, just outside your upper breastbone. "Feel for the tightness of the muscles," says Dr. Michael Reed Gach of the Acupressure Institute. Hold down both points, one on each side, with all of your fingers. Breathe very slowly and deeply, and keep your eyes closed while you hold the points, for two minutes, Dr. Gach adds.

Tackle your thumbs. The thumb area—the fleshy part at the base of your thumb, the thumb itself, and right at the base of the thumbnail—all contain acupressure trigger points for allergies and asthma. Take your time and massage your entire thumb for a few minutes, then switch to the other thumb, Dr. Gach says.

Take off your shoes. Give your feet a good rubdown, says Robert A. Edwards of the Somerset School of Massage Therapy. By giving yourself a foot massage, concentrating on the sides of your toes, you're bound to hit a couple reflexology points that may help relieve the problems of allergies and asthma.

Head for the trees. This may sound like the last thing you want to do when you have allergies. But the essential oils from fir and pine trees could improve your respiration. "These oils will help you drain congestion," says Michael Scholes of the Michael Scholes School of Aromatic Studies. You can emit these scents around your house or office by using different products such as diffusers and candles.

Breathing Lessons

You figure that you learned how to breathe the minute you were born. But you picked up some bad habits along the way, and that may contribute to breathing problems.

"Learning how to breathe more effectively can help your respiratory system in general and, as an extension, help with allergies and asthma", says yoga instructor Mara Carrico. Used with meditation and in yoga, proper breathing can help you relax and de-stress, an added bonus since stressful events can sometimes trigger an asthma attack. To counter or deflect this stress and calm the nervous system, Carrico advises her yoga students to breathe using the following techniques.

Breathe abdominally. When you inhale, expand your belly. When you exhale, draw your belly button in toward your spine by contracting your lower abdominals.

Keep the breaths long and equal. The idea is to make your inhalations the same length as your exhalations. For an even more relaxing effect, start to make your exhalations longer than your inhalations.

Breathe through your nose. If you are congested, this won't be easy, but give it a try. After practice, it should become easier, and you'll start to do it without noticing.

Of Mites and Men

The never-seen-but-often-felt dust mite lives in bedding and clothing. For many people, these microscopic spiderlike creatures pose no problem. In fact, no one is allergic to the dust mite. Instead, inhaling their droppings is what causes allergic symptoms. The little buggers aren't very easy to get rid of either. Although a weekly washing may get rid of the droppings, you have to wash your bedding in very hot water to kill the actual mites, says Euan R. Tovey, Ph.D., a research fellow at the Institute of Respiratory Medicine at the University of Sydney.

But Dr. Tovey and his colleagues have found the mite's kryptonite: eucalyptus oil. In a study by Dr. Tovey, washing clothes and bedding in eucalyptus oil killed off 95 percent of the dust mites in a wool blanket. To make a eucalyptus oil solution, mix one part dishwashing detergent, such as Sunlight, in three to five parts eucalyptus oil.

For a large washing machine, you will need a little less than a half-cup of this mixture. Start your machine, and when the bottom is covered with water, stop the machine. Then add a bit of this mix to the water. The mixture, after being added to the water, should stay milky for at least 10 minutes. After the 10 minutes are over, fill the washer, then add the rest of the mixture. Let your laundry soak for at least 30 minutes, and then wash as usual.

Dr. Tovey says that a eucalyptus oil washing once every two or three months will keep the mite population down and subsequently keep the mite's droppings down, as well. He still recommends washing your bedding—and that includes blankets, pillowcases, and comforters—in hot water once a week.

Colds and Flu

Natural Cures Are Nothing to Sneeze At

Colds and flus are America's most frequent illnesses, the cause of an estimated 650 million days of "limited activity" a year. That sounds like a lot, but it should probably be more: Doctors say that most of us don't rest enough when we get colds.

That's not the only thing that we've been doing wrong. When we get colds or the flu, many of us run to the doctor for antibiotics. And many physicians agree to write the prescriptions, even though antibiotics do nothing for these viral infections.

If ever there was an opportunity for holistic health care to come riding heroically to the rescue, this is it. Alternative practitioners have lots of solutions—solutions that actually work—for preventing and treating colds and flu.

Keeping Bugs at Bay

The best colds are the ones you don't get. Here are some suggestions for dodging the viral bullet.

Take echinacea. Boost your immune system herbally by taking echinacea at the first sign that a cold might be coming on. "It activates the specialized white blood cells that help destroy invading organisms such as cold viruses," says Dr. Varro E. Tyler of Purdue University School of Pharmacy and Pharmacal Sciences. Dr. Tyler recommends buying standard-ized tablets or capsules (available in most health food stores) and following the dosage directions carefully. Do not use echinacea for more than eight weeks at a time; if you have an autoimmune condition such as lupus, tuberculosis, or multiple sclerosis; or if you are allergic to chamomile, marigold, or other plants in the daisy family.

Grab a clove. Garlic is another of nature's great immunizers. Crush or mash a fresh clove or two into anything from pesto to salad dressing, or just eat half a clove three times a day. A more sociable option when you actually get a cold is to take garlic capsules. A typical dosage is 300 milligrams, three times a day, for as long as cold symptoms last, says Dr. Adriane Fugh-Berman of the Office of Alternative Medicine at the National Institutes of Health.

Drink water. It doesn't get any simpler than that, and yet keeping yourself hydrated with plenty of water—eight, eight-ounce glasses a day—is one of the simplest things you can do to beat a cold. That's because there are antibodies in your throat that can kill cold viruses, but getting dehydrated dries up the mucous membranes where those antibodies live, according to John Rogers, M.D., professor of family and community medicine at Baylor College of Medicine in Houston. If you do catch something, water even works as an expectorant for productive coughs. It also helps replenish lost fluids when a fever is burning you out.

Listen to the music. Most of us can sense when a cold is coming on. The next time that happens, fight back with music, says Dr. Steven Halpern of Inner Peace Music. When he feels his own immune system weakening, Dr. Halpern withdraws into a private room, puts on some soothing music, and repeats healing affirmations to himself ("I'm strong, I'm healthy" or variations on that theme). "Usually after five minutes, I can feel a difference in my stress level. By participating in my own self-healing process, I know that I'm contributing to the effectiveness of my recuperative powers," he says.

The Alternate Route to Recovery

No man is an island, which means that there's only so much insulation that you can put between yourself and the viruses that cause colds and flu. When the inevitable happens, here's what to do to minimize the damage.

Suck zinc. One of the more publicized health discoveries in the past few years has been the news that zinc disables colds like kryptonite zaps Superman. A study at the Cleveland Clinic Foundation found that 50 people with colds who sucked on lozenges laced with zinc every two hours reduced the duration of their symptoms by almost half.

If you're looking for zinc lozenges in the store, be careful to buy ones containing the same formula that was tested in Cleveland, zinc gluconate with glycine (marketed as Cold-Eeze). The effectiveness of other formulations on the market hasn't been proven by clinical trails.

Wear a wet T-shirt. We're talking about hydrotherapy here, not ogling. A basic principle of naturopathic medicine is to assist the body in its natural healing processes. In the case of a fever, Thomas Kruzel, N.D., a naturopathic physician in Portland, Oregon, and former president of the American Association of Naturopathic Physicians, suggests that you take a hot shower, soak a T-shirt in cold water, wring out as much water as possible, put it on, put on a dry wool or flannel shirt over it, and

---

Beating Back a Cold

When you feel like the Eighth Army used your body as a proving ground, start looking around for a grapefruit. "The first thing you should do is eat a lot of foods rich in vitamin C," says Laima Wesson, R.D., health educator-dietitian at the University of California, Los Angeles, student health service. "It's an antioxidant that helps strengthen your immune system." Citrus fruits and juices fit the bill here, as do red peppers, broccoli, and strawberries.

If your appetite has been lousy thanks to your cold, you can recharge your batteries with an easy-to-digest meal, like maybe a baked potato and a steaming bowl of soup. "Soups—especially tomato and vegetable soups—tend to be very rich in vitamin C, and they are a very palatable way of delivering nutrients," says Kris Clark, R.D., Ph.D., a nutritionist at Pennsylvania State University in University Park.

---

go to bed. "The idea," he says, "is to shock the white blood cells in your system into movement so that they can help fight the infection. The body tries to warm up the cold shirt, and that gets your blood circulating. It works extremely well."

Breathe in relief. For a stuffy head and blocked sinuses, Jeanne Rose of the Aromatic Plant Project suggests pouring some boiling water into a large heat-safe glass bowl. Add the following essential oils: one drop of rosemary, one drop of peppermint, and one drop of juniper berry. Allow the water to cool slightly. Put a towel over your head, bend over, and inhale the steam for a few minutes. Or you can put the bowl on the floor next to your bed, shut your bedroom door, and go to sleep. Essential oils are available in health food stores.

Cuts and Bruises

Ministering to Mishaps

Because cuts and bruises go back far longer than iodine and Band-Aids, organic remedies for coping with them abound. Here's a rundown of the essential elements needed to treat life's hard knocks.

Banishing the Bruises

Compress that contusion. When you bump your shin, the best way to reduce the swelling is to apply a little hydrotherapy. Immediately after the injury, start with some ice wrapped in a washcloth, says Dr. Thomas Kruzel of the American Association of Naturopathic Physicians. Leave the ice on for 10 to 15 minutes. You can repeat the treatment every two to four hours, or as needed for pain and swelling, he says.

After the swelling has gone down, alternate cold and hot compresses. For the hot part, soak a washcloth with hot tap water and hold it against the bruise for about three minutes. Switch to a wet washcloth wrapped around ice for a minute or so, and then return to the hot. Always start with the hot and end with the cold, alternating that process as many as three to five times. Wait for a few hours and repeat once or twice a day, says Dr. Kruzel.

Grab the green cube. A novel approach for chilling out a bruise is to use an ice cube filled with parsley. Parsley has long been a considered a remedy for dispelling black-and-blue marks, according to herbalist Sharleen Andrews-Miller, a faculty member at the

National College of Naturopathic Medicine in Portland, Oregon, and associate medicinary director at the college's public clinic. "Just whirl two handfuls of parsley in a blender or food processor with just enough water to make it look like slush," she says. Then pour the mixture in ice cube trays, filling them halfway, and freeze. When you get bruised, wrap the ice cubes in gauze or thin cloth and apply to the bruised spots. Apply them for 10 to 15 minutes, and repeat every two to four hours, as needed.

Get some internal protection. Eating oranges and grapefruits regularly can help bruises disappear faster and discourage their appearing in the first place, says retired botanist Dr. James A. Duke. That's because citrus fruits are rich in vitamin C and bioflavonoids, nutrients that help strengthen tiny blood vessels. That makes those vessels less prone to breakage and helps them heal more quickly. Try to add one or two citrus fruits as part of the recommended five or more servings of fruits and vegetables a day, differing them occasionally, says Dr. Duke.

Go to montana. Homeopaths tout the herb *Arnica montana* as a great cure for bruises.

Take it as soon as possible after an injury, says Jennifer Jacobs, M.D., assistant clinical professor of epidemiology at the University of Washington in Seattle and co-author of *Healing with Homeopathy*. Take the dosage listed on the package of the 12X, 30X, or 30C potencies, and repeat every hour for three doses, then twice a day until the pain and bruising subside, she says.

Topical ointments containing arnica are also available, according to Dr. Duke. Look for products containing up to 15 percent arnica oil, and follow the directions on the package. Homeopathic arnica products are available at health food stores.

Curing the Cuts

Don't forget the basics.

Certain traditions are worth keeping, including the basic steps you should take in treating wounds. These include applying direct but gentle pressure, if necessary, to stop any bleeding; washing the cut thoroughly with soap and water; and covering the cut with a bandage or other protection to keep the skin around it moist and to prevent further injury, says Dr. Kruzel.

Kill germs softly. Several varieties of natural products that will disinfect cuts naturally are available at health food stores. Dr. Duke's favorite is tea tree essential oil. He recommends diluting several drops of it in a couple of tablespoons of vegetable oil and applying it directly to the wound. If your skin gets irritated from the tea tree oil, try adding more vegetable oil.

Another effective natural antiseptic is calendula. To make a wash for treating cuts, pour a cup of boiling water over a teaspoon of dry calendula petals and steep for 10 minutes, Dr. Duke says. Allow it to cool until comfortably warm, then soak a clean cloth in the liquid and apply it as a compress on the wound. Calendula creams are available commercially, he adds, and are just as effective. Use them as directed on the package. If your skin isn't healing within three to five days, it is time to check with your doctor, suggests Dr. Duke.

Apply aloe. Products containing aloe vera are turning up everywhere these days, and for centuries, the sticky gel from inside the plant's leaves has been used to treat cuts and burns. The amount and quality of aloe vera in any commercial product varies widely, according to Dr. Varro E. Tyler of Purdue University School of Pharmacy and Pharmacal

---

Cuts above the Rest

There may come a time when a cut will need the judicious application of "suture therapy," otherwise known as getting stitches. How can you tell when you need stitches?

Any cut deep enough to show a rich yellow color needs stitches to heal properly. That yellow tint is a hint that the cut is into the layer of fat underneath the skin— too deep, in other words. If a cut shows white or flesh color, it's probably not very deep, and the remedies that our experts have outlined here can serve you well.

Here are some other instances when you'll want to seek out a doctor for cuts.

- The cut is deep or large (more than a half-inch long).
- The area is red, tender, inflamed, oozing, or discharging pus.
- You also have a fever or swollen lymph nodes.
- Cinders, gravel, or other foreign objects are lodged in the wound. You may need a doctor to numb the wound and clean it to prevent infection.

Sciences. Until standards are established, you can't be sure of what you're getting when you buy aloe products, he says. Your best bet is to keep an aloe plant handy and break off a leaf when needed. Squeeze out the pulp and apply it to the affected area.

Strengthen your system. If you cut yourself, Dr. Duke recommends drinking some echinacea tea to help ward off infection. Echinacea tea is available loose and in tea bags at health food stores. Do not use echinacea for more than eight weeks at a time; if you have an autoimmune condition such as lupus, tuberculosis, or multiple sclerosis; or if you are allergic to chamomile, marigold, or other plants in the daisy family.

Digestive Problems

You Don't Need to Gut It Out

From the second you bite into a pizza, that little chunk of cheese, dough, and tomato sauce begins a wild ride through the twists and turns that form your digestive system. Your esophagus pushes the food into your stomach, where acid burns and breaks it down into a gooey pulp. The remnants of that pizza make their way into your duodenum, a tube between your stomach and your intestines, where they get digested by even more chemicals. The souplike fodder crawls into and through the small intestine—all 20 feet of it—where most of the water and nutrients are absorbed. At the rate of two contractions an hour, the leftovers travel through the colon and end their journey through your body. You know the rest.

It's a complex system that requires all these different parts and processes working together. Most of the time, they do their jobs efficiently and rather uneventfully. But when something does go wrong, the whole system can be knocked out of whack. A problem with your stomach and esophagus heats up into heartburn. A snag in your intestines and colon brings about a number of problems—constipation, diarrhea, and irritable bowel syndrome. If you are like most people, you'll do anything to get the system up and running properly again.

Quieting the Internal Storm

Being the generation that invented the takeout burrito, it's not a surprise that we experience digestive woes. The number of over-the-counter remedies reflects our need for gastrointestinal relief. But you have other choices as well, choices that you may have never known about before. A mix of herbs, food, stress relief, and even some age-old acupressure can bring peace to your digestive process.

Fill up on fiber. Is constipation your problem? Eat fiber. Is irritable bowel syndrome bothering you? Eat more fiber. Is diverticulosis ticking you off? Get more fiber. Do you see a pattern here? "Fiber, fiber, and fiber are essential in preventing these problems," says Dr. Victor S. Sierpina of the University of Texas Medical Branch. Fiber keeps the digestive system on track. It bulks up the stool, making it quicker and easier for you to get rid of waste. That, in turn, helps you to avoid constipation, hemorrhoids, and diverticulosis—nasty little pouches that form along the colon walls.

If men ate the amount of fiber they should eat—about 25 to 30 grams a day—there would be almost no need for laxatives or other digestive medications, says Dr. Gene Spiller of the Health Research and Studies Center. Good sources of fiber include high-fiber cereal, whole grains, fruits (don't forget dried fruits, especially figs, prunes, and raisins), vegetables, and beans.

Supplement with psyllium. It seems contradictory, but this herbal supplement can help you with both constipation and diarrhea. Psyllium, a soluble fiber, absorbs a great deal of water and adds bulk to the stool, which helps with diarrhea. That increased bulk also speeds up the stool's travel time, which helps constipation. The digestive wonder supplement is also recommended for diverticulosis, hemorrhoids, and inflammatory bowel disease. You can find psyllium in the laxative section of supermarkets and drugstores in products like Metamucil. Take as directed on the package, Dr. Sierpina says.

Quell the burn. When you burn your skin, you reach for the aloe vera plant. The gel from inside the leaves soothes the burn. It can do the same to a heartburn fire raging inside your body as well, Dr. Sierpina says. Aloe vera juice cools heartburn and other indigestion problems by coating inflamed areas. You can find the drink in health food stores or herb stores. Follow package directions on how much to drink. Also, never use it for more than 8 to 10 days at a time.

Add some oils. Sometimes, your digestive system likes to go into a little spasm, contracting and moving at its own will without any regard for how you feel about it. Some essential oils might help put an end to your digestive muscles' cha-cha. The essential oils lavender and tarragon are thought to have antispasmodic qualities, which could help calm irate stomach and bowels, says Michael Scholes of the Michael Scholes School of Aromatic Studies. Dilute the essential oil by adding three or four drops of essential oil to ⅓ ounce of canola or sweet almond oil. Then rub the mixture in a circular motion around your abdominal and gastrointestinal region. If you are experiencing abdominal cramping, do this every half-hour until you feel a sense of relief.

Point to your problem. The ear bone is connected to the digestive system—at least in acupressure. Two different points inside your ear can help with digestive problems, says certified acupuncturist Dr. David Nickel. The first point helps balance your digestive system and is good for indigestion, nausea, belching, and heartburn. Press your finger in the shell of your ear one fingertip width up and back from the ear canal. Hold the point for five seconds, then release for five seconds. Continue with the five-second intervals for a minute, Dr. Nickel says. Inhale through your nose when you release the point. Exhale through your mouth when you apply the pressure.

Woods Lore

Many people know what it's like to have a bout of Montezuma's revenge while traveling in foreign lands. But what do you do when you find yourself in the jungles of Suriname in South America, miles from civilization? Look for the closest rediloksi tree. The Maroons, a people who have inhabited Suriname for four centuries, use the resin from inside the rediloksi tree to cure diarrhea, according to ethnobotanist Mark J. Plotkin, Ph.D., in his book *Tales of a Shaman's Apprentice*. They crush the resin and drink the powder with warm water.

But the tree resin also serves another important purpose to the people of the rain forest. When lit by a flame, the resin bursts into a clear blue fire and fills the air with the smell of pine. The Maroons use the resin to start a fire when it rains, because it burns more quickly than wet wood.

The second point creates elimination balance and helps with both constipation and diarrhea, Dr. Nickel says. This point is just above where the outer rim of your ear ends inside your ear. Again, hold the point for five seconds and then five seconds off, for a full minute.

Hold your ribs. "One of the most powerful points for helping yourself with digestive problems is located at the base of your rib cage," says Dr. Michael Reed Gach of the Acupressure Institute. Place your hands at the base of either side of your rib cage. Curve your fingers and press gradually upward and inward into the bottom of your rib cage, Dr. Gach says. Feel a niche or indentation. Hold that point for two minutes while you breathe slowly.

Strong-arm stomach problems. Two acupressure points on your arm can help relieve nausea, stomachaches, and indigestion, Dr. Gach says. The first point is in on the underside of your wrist. Bend your hand so that the crease between your hand and your arm appears. In the center of this crease is a small dip formed by your wrist bones. Hold your finger in the center of the crease for a minute or two using firm pressure as you breathe slowly and deeply.

The second point is about two inches higher than the first. Place your finger directly between the two bones in the underside of your forearm. It should be about three finger widths above the crease of your wrist. Sit comfortably as you press firmly for about two minutes.

Eat to the music. Put on some slow, calming music when it's time to eat. Whether you realize it or not, you probably eat to the beat. If you listen to a fast-paced metal selection or an up-tempo classical piece, you'll most likely shovel down the food. "You'll eat faster and take bigger bites. All of this could lead to indigestion," says Dr. Steven Halpern of Inner Peace Music.

"One of the ways I knew that the music I was composing was suitable for relaxation was to listen to it after eating a large meal. If I didn't experience indigestion and gas, I knew that it was conducive to relaxing the listener," says Dr. Halpern.

Calm the stomach and mind. It's not always a coincidence that your stomach sends you hate mail during a stressful event like a big meeting or a fight. Stress triggers some digestive problems, especially irritable bowel disease. And stress makes any digestive ailment worse. Once you feel the problem arise, you start to panic, which makes your digestive muscles contract and act up even more.

But with a little imagery, you can break the cycle, says Dr. Larry J. Feldman of the Pain and Stress Rehabilitation Center. During an episode, picture yourself on a beach. Feel the sand, hear the seagulls and the crashing of the waves, and smell the salty ocean air, says Dr. Feldman. Do this for a couple minutes, or until you feel better. This quick and easy exercise may be all that you need to cut off your stress

response and help bring ease to your digestive problem sooner.

Go against your gut feeling. This technique is an antidote and has your mind trying to outsmart your stomach. Choose a word that describes what you are feeling. Let's say that you have heartburn. You choose the word *hot*. Then think of a word that is the direct opposite of that. You would pick *cool*. Keep repeating that word and try really hard to actually feel the word. Using your mind, you can bring relief to the rest of your body, Dr. Feldman says.

Time for Tea

When your stomach rumbles more than a California earthquake, you probably don't want to consume anything stronger than a cup of tea. But tea may be the strongest thing you can swallow down for your problems. Several herbal teas can come to your aid for various digestive problems, Dr. Sierpina says. Try one or several of the following herbal teas the next time your stomach and digestive system act up. General instructions for proper use of these teas is to steep a teaspoon of the herb for 10 minutes in boiling water. Sip a cup three times a day. Many packaged herbal teas come with product directions, in which case it's best to follow them.

General stomach upset: Use peppermint, spearmint, or blackberry. Also go with the old standby chamomile.

Colitis and other inflammation problems: Use licorice root tea, slippery elm bark, or goldenseal.

Nausea: A ginger tea can quell the queasiest of stomachs. "Ginger is great for nausea," Dr. Sierpina says. If you have some serious nausea, try Dr. Sierpina's homemade concoction, which sounds like it would make you queasy: Mix a half-cup of ginger ale, a half-cup of green tea, a teaspoon of honey, a teaspoon of grated ginger, and lemon juice to flavor.

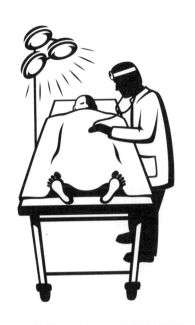

Quest for the Best

They're the best in their fields. And they got that way, in part, by using the best remedies around—the natural kind. Learn how these men unleashed their own personal healing power.

You Can Do It!

They may be ordinary guys, but they've tapped into some extraordinary methods for healing all of their ills. They've taken charge of their own health. You can, too.

Part Five

Real-Life Scenarios

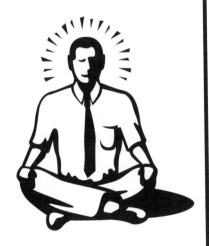

Quest for the Best They're the best in their fields.
And they got that way, in part, by using the best remedies around—the natural kind. Learn how these men unleashed their own personal healing power.

Michael Tucker, Actor

From Hollywood Actor to Devoted Husband

The actor Michael Tucker believes that he experienced a minor medical miracle, thanks to what may be the most pleasurable of all of the alternative therapies.

He discovered during his annual checkup that his cholesterol had dropped from a dangerously high reading of 240 to a quite respectable 176. Since he hadn't changed his diet significantly, or his modest commitment to exercise, he'd expected less pleasant news. What accounted for this dramatic improvement?

"I have no medical explanation," he says, "other than the fact that my level of stress is at an all-time low."

And why is that?

"I think it's because I make love to my wife at least twice a day," Tucker says.

The healing power of sex doesn't seem to be an especially unusual or uncomfortable topic of conversation for Michael Tucker, who for eight very successful years played nice-guy attorney Stuart Markowitz on the prime-time TV series *L.A. Law.* The real-life spouse with whom he shares his conjugal intimacies, Jill Eikenberry, starred as Markowitz's wife, Ann Kelsey, on the series.

Perhaps Tucker's open-

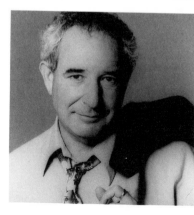

ness on sexual subjects is fitting for a couple whose characters had legions of viewers speculating during one memorable season about what the sexual technique known as the Venus Butterfly might be. There's nothing to snicker at, though, about Tucker's interest in Tantra, an Eastern discipline designed to enhance sex both physically and spiritually. Through his training in Tantra and many other courses, seminars, and studies on communication, sexuality, and intimacy, Tucker says that he has utterly redefined his relationship with his wife.

That Tucker would find Tantra spiritually uplifting makes perfect sense since Tantra is based on a series of ancient Hindu teachings that are aimed at accomplishing just that goal. Tantra teaches that lovemaking can be a form of meditation and a vehicle to a higher state of consciousness. One of its guiding principles is that men can learn to control their ejaculations, thereby prolonging the sex act indefinitely. The union of male and female during sex is seen as a way of connecting to cosmic forces of tremendous transformative power.

Tucker doesn't doubt for a moment that such a transformation is possible, because he has experienced it himself. "There are times during intimacy when it feels as if Jill and I are in an elevated state of being," he says. "We get high from this. There are a lot of ways to get high, but this is the best I've ever found."

His training in Tantra and the many other courses the couple have taken helped Tucker to recognize that popular U.S. culture teaches men to harbor selfish and self-defeating views of sex. "We have the whole direction of this thing backward," he says. "I'm definitely a pleasure-seeking missile, with food and sex and every other form of gratification. I chased my own pleasure for years. But all of them always left me vaguely dissatisfied, and I couldn't figure out why. What I learned when I began studying Tantra is that the reason I was vaguely dissatisfied is that satisfying my own pleasure is not what I really want. I don't want a woman servicing me. I want to give my woman what she really wants and then be acknowledged for it."

Some of Tucker's thoughts on the subject go decidedly against the all-American, John Wayne school of masculine self-sufficiency. In particular, Tantra places an emphasis on pleasing the woman that some men may find unduly subservient. Tucker is not among them. To the contrary, he's convinced that Tantra teaches a truer style of male power. "I think that every man wants to be a hero for his woman," he says. "He wants to give her safety and security as well as pleasure. He wants to deliver her love. And when we do it, we don't feel vaguely dissatisfied at all. We feel like a million bucks."

Tucker first encountered the world of alternative medicine during his years in Hollywood. His wife first encouraged him to accompany her to a seminar on meditation being taught by the famous New Age guru, Deepak Chopra, M.D., executive director of the Chopra Center for Well-Being in La Jolla, California. "I was totally skeptical," he says. But he came away impressed, despite himself.

Tucker began meditating daily, which, in turn, made him receptive to trying other forms of alternative therapy. "The meditation definitely keyed me in to the fact that there was more about myself than I knew," he says.

Another major impetus for Tucker's alternative journey was his wife's bout with breast cancer. The disease was diagnosed almost simultaneously with their being cast in *L.A. Law*, and the two spent their first season on the hit

series wondering whether Eikenberry would recover. She did, but the experience helped convince Tucker and Eikenberry that enjoying life was not something they could postpone until some undefined point in the future.

By the time *L.A. Law* ended its run in 1994, Tucker and Eikenberry were prepared to more or less drop out of the Hollywood rat race. "It was as if we had achieved everything we thought we wanted at the same time that Jill got cancer," he recalls. "We looked at each other and said that's not what we want. We want more." They sold their house in southern California and moved to Mill Valley, a wooded suburb north of San Francisco.

Holistic health care now appears to be completely and seamlessly integrated into the couple's lives. Tucker sees a Chinese medicine practitioner on occasion—acupuncture cleared up a cyst on his shoulder that was pinching a nerve—and both he and Eikenberry use homeopathic remedies regularly. The couple devotes much of their time and energy to giving lectures and leading workshops on surviving breast cancer and deepening relationships. Eikenberry is also involved in the Women's Leadership Organization, which runs seminars on women's fulfillment. Acting is not a priority.

In the years they've been out on the lecture circuit, Tucker has noticed that the doctors they meet have a much different attitude toward alternative medicine than they used to. "You wouldn't believe how different the conversation is now," he says. "They're all talking about acupuncture and visualization—stuff they would have scoffed at a few years ago."

He's a firm believer in the idea of complementary medicine, and envisions a day in which conventional and alternative therapists will work side by side, each referring patients to the other. The goal of health care, Tucker believes, needs to be broadened beyond its current focus on curing disease.

"Wellness is much more than just the absence of sickness," he says. "It's a far more elevated position, closely akin to bliss."

Tom Harkin, U.S. Senator

Leading the Fight in Congress

Prominently displayed on the wall of Senator Tom Harkin's office in Washington, D.C., is the famous photograph of the Chinese student dissident facing down a tank during the Tiananmen Square uprising of 1989. The picture tells you a lot about the senator's battles to have alternative medicine taken seriously in the Capitol's corridors of power. It also tells you a lot about how this populist politician from Iowa likes to picture himself.

Sen. Harkin, a Democrat, was the driving force behind the creation of the Office of Alternative Medicine (OAM). Established in 1992 as an arm of the National Institutes of Health (NIH), it has been a veritable volcano of controversy ever since. The OAM's job, in Sen. Harkin's view, is to "fully investigate and validate" various types of alternative medicine. This was not, it turned out, a mandate that the NIH felt comfortable assuming.

"The internal structure of the NIH fought me every step of the way," Sen. Harkin says. "They said that researching alternative medicine was 'junk science.' Or they claimed that there was already some kind of study going on at the NIH. They had all kinds of bureaucratic reasons. The real reason is that too many scientists today are locked into a rigid way of thinking that doesn't leave room for investigating unconventional approaches."

Political Change

Like many people who become passionate about alternative medicine, Sen. Harkin's interests grew out of personal experience—three of them, in

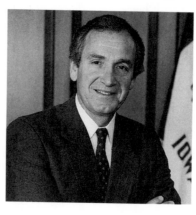

his case. The first came in 1990 when he was approached by a former colleague, Berkley Bedell, who was suffering simultaneously from Lyme disease and prostate cancer. Bedell had resigned from his seat in the U.S. House of Representatives to fight the diseases, Sen. Harkin says. Despite his wealth and connections, the former congressman found few reliable resources that could tell him anything about possible treatments outside of mainstream medicine. The government should be doing more, he told his old friend from Iowa, to make such information available.

Sen. Harkin was convinced at that encounter that Bedell would soon die. "I told my wife, 'I think I've seen Berkley for the last time,'" he recalls. Instead, Bedell triumphed over his illnesses with the help of highly controversial therapies.

As it happened, at about the same time, Sen. Harkin was presiding over hearings in which advocates of alternative medicine testified about the lack of federally funded research into unconventional therapies. The combination of the two experiences led Sen. Harkin to seek, and win, an appropriation of $2 million to start the OAM. Harkin's belief that alternative therapies were worth investigating was soon to be underscored by a more direct encounter.

He had long suffered from allergies, an annual affliction that had grown steadily worse over the years. The number of antihistamines that he ingested increased just as steadily. After sneezing his way through a meeting with Bedell, his old friend encouraged him to meet a man who claimed to have an answer: bee pollen therapy.

Sen. Harkin was soon taking bee pollen and feeling much better. His resolve to keep the OAM up and running deepened.

It deepened further with Sen. Harkin's third personal experience with alternative medicine, this one the most powerful of all. His brother developed thyroid cancer, and the tumors were causing him substantial pain. A doctor who knew of Sen. Harkin's involvement with the OAM suggested that an acupuncturist he knew might help. He did. "My brother was a smart guy, an M.B.A., an engineer, all that kind of stuff," Sen. Harkin says. "He couldn't believe how much those treatments relieved his pain."

Growing Pains

Despite his identification with the Tiananmen Square protester, Sen. Harkin is hardly a powerless figure in Washington, D.C. First elected to the Senate in 1984 after a decade in the House of Representatives, he accumulated sufficient seniority to become chairman of the powerful Senate Appropriations Subcommittee that oversees funding for the U.S. Department of Health and Human Services, which runs the NIH.

Thanks in part to Sen. Harkin's support, the OAM's annual budget increased steadily to a peak of $20 million in fiscal year 1998. That money has helped finance a series of studies that are investigating ways in which various alternative approaches might be brought to bear on everything from AIDS and depression to asthma and cancer.

None of this has come easily. Besides the resistance he encountered from the NIH leadership, Sen. Harkin found himself locked in a divisive battle with the first director of the OAM itself. Joseph Jacobs, M.D., was chosen as the ideal person to bridge the gap between alternative and conventional medicines. It didn't work out that way. Dr. Jacobs resigned after 24 stormy months in office, accusing Sen. Harkin and his allies of being more interested in promoting alternative therapies than in researching their value objectively.

The power struggle between the senator and the director generated considerable press, much of it unfavorable to Sen. Harkin. It was written that "the OAM is widely perceived by those in the medical mainstream as an unscientific organization that has been captured by the alternative medicine lobby."

Sen. Harkin didn't back down, though. Instead, he upped the ante, initiating a campaign to increase the OAM's authority so that it could fund its own research studies without going through the NIH bureaucracy. And Wayne Jonas, M.D., one of the country's leading experts on—and advocates for—homeopathy, was appointed as the new director of the OAM.

One development that has cheered Sen. Harkin as these battles have stretched on is the growing acceptance of alternative medicine that he finds among his colleagues. More and more senators and congressmen, he says, have experienced the healing power of various alternative therapies in their own lives, either for themselves or for their families. He's convinced that, in this respect, Washington only mirrors an ever-growing acceptance of alternative methods by the American public as a whole.

"For too long, we've had a system of medicine in America in which the attitude was always, 'The doctor knows best,'" he says. "Well, I think a lot of people are saying, 'I'm not so sure about that.' They're saying, 'Maybe if I can listen to my body and really think and learn about what's happening to me, maybe I can make some of my own choices.'"

Contrary to the way some people view him, Sen. Harkin says that he's not a zealot who believes that alternative medicine will magically cure any and every illness. He has recommended bee pollen therapy to lots of people, he says. Some it has helped; others it hasn't. Nor does he have an ax to grind against conventional medicine. He feels that there's value in both approaches.

"I believe that in my lifetime—and hopefully I have another 20 years left, at least—you're going to see a merging into a fully complementary medical system," he says. "Younger doctors are coming along who aren't as rigid as a lot of the older ones are."

Kevin Overland, Olympic Medalist

Some Needling Saved His Olympics

Just weeks before the 1998 Winter Olympics, Kevin Overland's coaches and trainers stood around him, telling him that he probably wasn't going to make it to Nagano, Japan. The speed skater had suffered a terrible muscle tear near his groin, and his coaches and trainers said that only time—and a good deal of it—would heal the wound.

But time was the one thing Overland didn't have. In order to make the Olympics, he had to skate the very next weekend at the trials, or else the Canadian Olympic speed skating team was going to leave him behind—again.

Four years earlier, a 19-year-old Overland was poised to compete in the 1994 Olympics. But two weeks before the Olympic trials, he was in a car accident and suffered whiplash—ending his chances of competing that year. So here he was again, weeks before the Olympics with an injury that would probably keep him from the games. "I was in an utter panic. I had all of these flashbacks of the car accident in 1994. I thought maybe the Olympics weren't in it for me," he says. He would be starting a regimen of physical therapy, but he knew that conventional therapy alone wouldn't heal him in time to compete.

A friend suggested—actually insisted—that Overland visit an acupuncturist. "I went into it very skeptical. I didn't believe in all this mystical stuff, but I wasn't in a position to be negative about it. So I went," Overland says.

Only days after he was practically written off for the Olympics, Overland skated in two 500-meter races, one 1000-meter race, and one 1500-meter

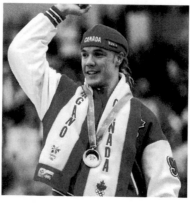

race. He qualified for the Olympics in all three events. More than that, he was just shy of the world record in the 1000-meter. "I was racing like I wasn't hurt. I truly believe that without the acupuncture, I wouldn't have been able to do it," he says.

Not only did he manage to qualify, but Overland continued on to the 1998 Winter Olympics, where he won a bronze medal in the 500-meter race.

Now a True Believer

Overland says that his miraculous recovery is all the proof he needs to believe in the ancient Chinese medical art. He refers the skeptics to a teammate of his who suffered the same injury that fateful weekend. That skater took the traditional physical therapy route, while Overland used physical therapy in combination with acupuncture. His friend didn't make it to Nagano. Overland did. "People want to see results and data? He wasn't able to go, and I was," he says.

During his recovery time, Overland went to his acupuncturist, Kevin Elander, almost every day. Besides the needle treatment, he also followed other aspects of Traditional Chinese Medicine. He took the prescribed internal and external elixirs—herbal combinations intended to improve blood circulation, help lung function, and keep the kidneys healthy. He also took the herb ginseng as an overall tonic.

The therapy focused on the skater's injury in two ways. First, it controlled the pain so that Overland could compete, even though he had not completely healed. "It allowed me to do what I had to do to get by," he says.

Second, using acupuncture helped speed up the healing time. It is believed that acupuncture affects the nervous system and triggers the release of neurochemicals that naturally relieve pain and inflammation. By the time he reached Nagano, Overland says, he felt almost completely better. But his acupuncturist also worked on another aspect of the Olympian as well—his brain. "I was stressed out of my mind," he says. The acupuncture helped refocus Overland's energy and control his stress.

To keep up with his acupuncture treatment in Nagano, Overland found another acupuncturist right outside the Olympic village: local practitioner Susumu Koyama. As soon as he examined Overland, Koyama knew exactly what his injury was (even though Overland didn't tell him) and continued the treatment. Word got around, and soon Koyama was treating roughly 20 different competitors from the Olympic village as well as entertaining questions from other doctors and the Western media about this "new" treatment. Meanwhile, Overland finished third in the 500-meter sprint and found himself on the podium, accepting the bronze medal for his country after skating what he called "the best race of my whole career."

His recovery mystified his trainers and coaches. "I feel like I have discovered a gem. It is such a great way to heal," he says. The Canadian speed skating team massage therapist, whom Overland also credits with his speedy recovery, took the time to learn acupressure—a similar form of Chinese medicine that triggers key points with touch instead of needles. As a result, the team had access to some form of the technique while they were in Nagano. Overland says that everyone on the team was impressed with its results in helping athletes cope with injury and pain, without resorting to drugs.

Since then, Overland has converted some other athletes to using acupuncture. His sister Cindy, also a speed skater on the Canadian team, now uses the ancient technique. His girlfriend, Dutch speed skater Marianne

Timmer, tried it in Nagano to help with a lower-back injury that had been nagging her for awhile. She went on to win two gold medals. "She can't explain how her lower-back pain went away except that the only thing she did different this time was the acupuncture," he says.

Part of the Routine

Overland now uses acupuncture on a regular basis and whenever he suffers an injury. "Let's put it this way, I go to the acupuncturist before I go to the therapist now. That's bold," he says.

But he doesn't forsake the traditional physical therapy. He says that the two work extremely well together and should complement each other. "There are different ways to heal things. Acupuncture is definitely a route to explore. I highly suggest it to people who are stuck with an injury that won't go away," he says.

Thanks to his success in Nagano, Overland has found himself somewhat of a star in his home country of Canada and around the world. "Life has changed dramatically in Holland and Europe for me. Over there, speed skating is a superstar sport. I am on talk shows all the time," he says. A Dutch software company now sponsors Overland, taking some pressure off him financially. He now trains part of the year in Holland and is already setting his sights on the 2002 Winter Olympics in Salt Lake City.

In the meantime, he'll continue to train and take advantage of all the perks and pleasantries that go along with being an Olympic medal winner. And he'll keep his acupuncture treatments going as well. "I can't avoid that fact that acupuncture was the make-me-or-break-me factor before the Olympics," he says. "I would never have even thought about it unless someone suggested it to me. Am I ever glad I did it."

Oscar Janiger, M.D., Alternative Healing Author and Expert

An Alternative Pioneer

After years of seeking out alternative treatments for his patients, Dr. Oscar Janiger still found himself banging his head against the medical mainstream's proverbial wall: Real medical doctors don't use holistic medicine, he heard over and over again.

But the professor of psychiatry at the University of California, Irvine, California College of Medicine had a theory. He believed that these real medical doctors *did* use alternative medicine but that the medical community's mood kept them from going public with it. To prove his theory, he and his associates interviewed hundreds of doctors around the United States.

The interviews revealed that a number of traditional doctors practiced—or were at least open to—alternative healing. But the interviews also proved what Dr. Janiger suspected: that many classically trained medical doctors used holistic treatment on themselves but not on their patients. "One doctor said that he used a chiropractor all the time himself, but he'd never say a word about it to his patients," he says.

An element of fear kept these doctors from publicly admitting that they used alternative remedies. It also kept many of them from passing their wisdom on to their patients. Many thought that they would gain reputations as weirdos and that they would be treated as outcasts in the medical community.

Yet all these people didn't know that the same colleagues they feared reprisals from also used alternative medicine. It was time to stand up

and be counted, Dr. Janiger says. "We needed some facts to establish if their fears were real or imagined," he says. Using the results of the survey, he co-wrote *A Different Kind of Healing: Doctors Speak Candidly about Their Success with Alternative Medicine.* The book shed light on the fact that fellow traditionally trained medical experts were partaking in, and finding success with, alternative healing.

In his book, Dr. Janiger detailed the alternative practices these doctors used. One doctor used aloe vera for burns and bug bites and even gargled with it to help relieve sore throats. Another doctor used chamomile tea for anxiety and insomnia, and one even used it for conjunctivitis. Another used a folk technique that he got from his Turkish parents. For a big bruise, he'd make an onion poultice and leave it on all night. By morning, the bruise was well on its way to being healed.

Searching for Better Options

Years before the study and the book were even conceived, Dr. Janiger says that he was on a quest for alternative options for his patients. "I felt somewhat dissatisfied with the treatment choices I had with conventional and mainstream medicine. I had some creative ideas that looked elsewhere," he says.

He especially felt that there had to be more for people with chronic conditions.

So Dr. Janiger headed out into the world

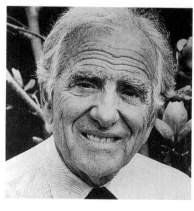

to find these ways. He studied with healers in the Amazon. He learned about Chinese medicine, herbs, and chiropractic medicine. He found other medical professionals who wanted to look outside the barriers of the medical establishment. In the early 1970s, Dr. Janiger accepted an appointment as chairman of the research committee of the Holmes Center for Research in Holistic Healing, a nonprofit foundation that provided grants for the scientific investigation of unconventional medical practices. Through actual scientific research, the organization hoped to legitimize holistic medicine, Dr. Janiger says. As one of the first organizations to give out money for the study of alternative medicine, they were swamped by requests and proposals.

Over the course of 10 years, Dr. Janiger and the organization awarded tens of thousands of dollars for the study of alternative and holistic medicine. "We funded some of the most outstanding men and women who couldn't get the money elsewhere. There were no sources for alternative funds whatsoever," he says. One of the early grants went to a young doctor named Dean Ornish, who went on to world renown for his study of the effects of lifestyle on heart disease.

The Holmes Center also acted as a clearinghouse and education center for the study and practice of alternative medicine. The group had power, Dr. Janiger believes, because it was a collection of well-respected, qualified medical doctors and nurses from all over the country. "It was a very prestigious group all believing in this one thing. . . . I think we were a force in getting this alternative medicine movement off the ground," he says.

Despite his reputable background, Dr. Janiger says that his reputation back then was on "shaky ground" because of his interest in alternative medicine. He credits the rise of alternative medicine into the mainstream with the early efforts of himself and his friends at the Holmes Center. "We kindled some of this, and then we let the fires burn," he says. It was his work at the center that spawned the idea of a poll of traditional doctors and their use of holistic treatments.

In his eighties, Dr. Janiger still practices medicine and recommends many alternative remedies to his patients. For chronic migraine patients, for example, he advises hydrotherapy—the use of hot and cold water to heal. He also has several patients taking the herb St.-John's-wort for their depression. "I had one patient whom no other antidepressant helped. But he has been on St.-John's-wort for six months, and he's better," he says. Dr. Janiger has never had a patient turn down a holistic or alternative treatment.

A Marriage of Medicines

Dr. Janiger doesn't dismiss his traditional medical training in favor of alternative healing. In fact, in many cases, he says, Western methods of medicine are the only options doctors have. But medical professionals should be open to using all avenues of healing. "This doesn't mean that alternative medicine is necessarily better than regular medicine. We're talking about an understanding between the two that allows the best of both to be used," he says.

A traditional doctor doesn't have to embrace everything associated with alternative medicine. "You don't have to bury an onion under a rock during a full moon or anything. You can just do innovative things in general according to your liking."

The perfect example of how traditional and alternative medicine should work together occurred when Dr. Janiger was in the jungle studying the ancient healing arts of a shaman—a member of a tribal society who acts as a medium between the visible world and an invisible spirit world and who also practices magic or sorcery for the purpose of healing. After following him around for a week, Dr. Janiger noticed that the shaman had developed bronchitis. Through an interpreter, Dr. Janiger asked if he could give the shaman a shot of penicillin. The shaman smiled and cheerfully accepted by pulling down his pants so that Dr. Janiger could give him the shot. A few days later, the shaman was better.

As Dr. Janiger's expedition drew to a close, he asked the interpreter to tell the shaman that he hoped that he hadn't offended him by offering his Western medicine. The shaman smiled and replied, "Tell him that if he believes in my medicine, I'll believe in his."

You Can Do It! They may be ordinary guys, but they've tapped into some extraordinary methods for healing all of their ills. They've taken charge of their own health. You can, too.

Open to Alternatives

Michael Gould, Melbourne, Florida

Date of birth: August 15, 1949

Profession: International economic developer

It can be hard to maintain a healthy lifestyle with my irregular schedule and all the places I have to go. But I force myself to do it. Wherever I am, I make sure that I walk every day. I just take some meditation tapes and walk for 30 to 40 minutes before I get into a suit and tie. My philosophy is to allow time for myself first. You feel the results all day when you do that.

I also use herbs to keep me on an even keel. Every day, I take calming herbs like skullcap and valerian. I tend to be kind of high-strung, so I take valerian to keep me calm and peaceful, St.-John's-wort to make me happy, and hawthorn to keep my heart strong. My blood pressure tends to be a little high, but I think the hawthorn does wonders for keeping it down.

I first got interested in herbs through my study of Native American philosophy—that and the fact that my wife, Kathleen, and I share a belief in their value. Kathleen owns an herb shop, and I like to go there and drink all kinds of tea. If something is bothering me, I can go right to the shop to take care of it. Kathy gives me herbs all the time; I take them right there.

When I'm at home in Florida, one of the gifts I have is free time and some relaxation. When I travel, I'm more prone to stress, and I try to shield myself from this stress. I visually surround myself with a white light, and I say,

"I am not going to let myself be affected by negative influences today."

Even adjusting to the weather in different places can be hard. In the winter, I have to travel a lot between Florida and cities in the north, so I use herbs to help me adjust to the climate changes. I take astragalus, shizandra, and mullein, and immune-enhancing herbs.

Working in sales involves so much inter-action with other people. I deal with that upper 5 percent of the population who have a lot of money—a lot of type A personalities. So I try to use calming ways in my business. I'm very conscious of the psychological side of interacting with people. I believe that we're all one, and that helps me stay calm and focused. And I don't look at sales as being goal-oriented. I think that you have to give things over to the universe and it will all take care of itself.

I learned something years ago that really helps. When I meet people of other nationalities, I visualize stepping out of my body to observe the scene before me. I try to take my ego out of the situation so that I'm not trying to influence events. This helps me look more objectively at people from other cultures. Many people in sales try to take over the situation, but it's much easier to sell something if you look at the customer's perspective, not your own. I try to give information rather than opinions. I think I learned to do this because I've always had an interest in different philosophies.

My exercise philosophy matches my lifestyle as a whole. My family lives on the beach, and so my wife and I walk there every day and then go to the gym three days a week. I'm not into jogging really hard or doing things like that. My exercise, like everything else, I try to do in a calming way.

Don't Poke Fun at Acupuncture

Ben Pisano, Cos Cob, Connecticut

Date of birth: February 6, 1941

Profession: Stonemason

When you don't feel good, you never hurt your back. You're more careful then. It's when your back feels great that you're not careful and an injury happens.

I've been a stonemason all of my adult life. I learned a little bit of the trade before I left my home in southern Italy in 1959. I was 18 and came to the United States as a "greenhorn." Now I have my own company: My brother and I are partners, and we have two or three guys working with us. But I still do a lot of the physical masonry work.

I've hurt my back many times. I don't know if my work caused it, but one thing leads to another and maybe being a stonemason has something to do with it. Back problems sometimes go away on their own . . . just with time passing. You stay at home and rest; eventually, it gets better. When it wouldn't, I tried using a heating pad, lying down on the floor (because that's the most comfortable place when your back really hurts), taking aspirin. Finally, I started going to chiropractors. Actually, I went to a lot of them. I'd see them for a month or five weeks before I could go back to work, and then for another three to four months after that. I felt like I was going every minute, and I still didn't feel better. It never helped.

In the winter of 1997, I hurt so bad that I couldn't even lift my leg off the floor one inch. The doctors said that I had herniated disks and that I might need surgery. Then one day, my friend Tony said, "Why don't you go see Babs Meade? I'm a patient of hers, and she's gonna fix you up with acupuncture." Tony's a good friend of mine. He's a landscape architect, and we do a lot of work together. So I trust him.

Needle Me

Tony said that Babs would put needles in my back, give me massages—things like that.

I didn't know how it would feel, but I wasn't scared. When you have a lot of pain, you're not scared of anything. You just want to feel better. I'd probably be scared if I was feeling *good* and someone said, "I'm going to poke some needles in your back."

When I went for my first treatment that winter, I could hardly move at all. Bending to put on my socks was impossible. Babs did massage and acupuncture, which released the muscle spasms in my back. Then I went home and lay down on the floor. Later that night, I got up off the floor—just like that. No problem. The improvement was dramatic. I'm not saying that it will always happen this way, but this time, "Wow!"

While my back was the worst, I went for acupuncture treatments a couple times a week. Babs put about 20 or 30 needles in my back, my fingers, toes, head, ears. The needles are small, and she leaves them there for about 20 minutes. Then she takes them out and massages your back. Sometimes she uses a special massage oil. And she has soft music playing to help you relax.

Now I go about once every five weeks for massage and acupuncture, even though I'm not in pain. It makes my back feel good, and it will prevent the back spasms that made my life miserable that winter.

Play Ball

How well has it worked? I play in a boccie league in Stamford. During the summer, we play a couple times a week. Many other years, I couldn't play because of my back. Now, after acupuncture, I almost never miss a game.

Acupuncture helped me when I felt the worst and keeps me feeling good. I would definitely say to anyone with back pain (or any other kind of pain), "Try it." Go ahead and go. It really works.

Winning the Fight of My Life

Jim Rindock,
Allentown, Pennsylvania

Date of birth: April 27, 1952

Profession: Postal worker

"No evidence of residual or recurrent tumor." After 2½ years of waging an all-out war on my cancer, those seven words printed on a white postcard were like a trumpet signaling that the tumor had finally retreated. The cancer was completely gone. My wife cried at the news. I was in shock. It took several days and a reassurance call to my doctor before I felt the weight of the cancer lifted from my shoulders.

The fight of my life began with what I thought were severe sinus headaches. The pain was so intense I thought my face was going to fall off. Then on New Year's Day 1995, I had a seizure and was rushed to the hospital. That's when they discovered that I had cancer. The prognosis wasn't good. It was an aggressive kind of tumor called astrocytoma. The doctors said that it was in an advanced stage and was probably terminal. They performed emergency surgery to remove as much of the tangerine-sized tumor as possible. That was just the beginning of my fight.

I was determined to do everything in my power to beat the cancer—for myself and for my wife and three children. I underwent 37 radiation treatments, two rounds of chemotherapy, and two experimental injections of monoclonal antibodies. But none of this heavy artillery shrank the tumor. That's when I launched a new plan of attack: I began trying alternative therapies.

Before the cancer, I laughed at alternative medicine. I thought it was bizarre. But when you have cancer, you'll try anything. If someone had told me that jumping off a roof would cure my cancer, I would have done it.

I went on a supplement regimen to strengthen my immune system. I took vitamin C, garlic, cow cartilage, and something called Bio-Immunozyme Forte. I drank an herbal tea every day, inhaled the aroma of frankincense every night, went for regular massages and counseling sessions, and began going to church every week. Each day, I would imagine myself shooting laser bullets at the tumor. It was as if I could actually hear the tumor exploding.

I think that the key weapon in my war against cancer, though, was the strict macrobiotic diet of organic fruits, vegetables, whole grains, and beans. After about three months of being on the diet, the tumor began to shrink.

Because my doctors and I aren't sure which of the therapies worked, I have continued most of them to be on the safe side. I did relax my diet quite a bit, and that may be to blame for a tiny remnant tumor that showed up in January. They attacked the problem with a special kind of neurosurgery, and my prognosis remains positive. That scare was enough to get me back on the strict diet and to teach me that I may have won the battle, but to win the war I have to stick with the alternative therapies for the long haul.

I've been back at work separating mail since October 1997. I work for five hours and then take a nap before the kids return from school. I'm still fatigued and sometimes have short-term memory loss, but I've gained back the 40 pounds I had lost. My co-workers donated their vacation days to make up for the months that I was unable to work. My friends held a prayer vigil and ran fund-raisers to help pay for the alternative therapies, which cost about $250 a month and are not covered by my health insurance.

There's a saying: An individual gets cancer; it takes a community to beat cancer. In my case, it took an army of doctors, family, friends, and co-workers to win the first major battle. The war may not be quite over yet, but when I get rid of the cancer this time, I'm not going to give it a chance to come back.

Yes to Yoga

Les Lang,
Chapel Hill, North Carolina

Date of birth: July 15, 1941

Profession: Medical writer

Perhaps my job as a medical writer has made me a slight hypochondriac, but I've always considered myself a relatively health-conscious guy. Back in 1978, at the tender age of 36, I jogged regularly, I loved playing basketball and softball, and I watched what I ate. And after reading a bit on Eastern philosophy and hearing a friend constantly rave about the benefits of yoga, my curiosity peaked and I decided to give it a try.

After a few hatha yoga lessons, I could understand my friend's enthusiasm. I became an immediate devotee and began taking classes once a week and practicing regularly at home.

The reason for my instant devotion was the class's slow individualized focus. To begin the class, the instructor would have us sit quietly on the floor and concentrate on our breathing. Then, a series of gradual and gentle stretches and breathing exercises would be introduced. The postures eventually became more aerobic and challenging as you progressed. The class usually ended with a "dead pose," where you're lying on your back, arms slightly extended and legs spread, while your breathing returns to normal.

A Lifetime Pursuit

I think that any yoga teacher will tell you that doing yoga is a lifelong process. As I become more fossilized chronologically, I realize that you really must follow up with occasional classes because your postures may need to be corrected. I'm lucky because I married a yoga instructor, Barbara, back in 1980.

Sometimes, Barbara and I practice double yoga, which is simply yoga postures done in pairs. One such posture is called a bridge, and it requires each person to support the other. I think that it's a fun way to practice yoga and great at enhancing your romantic relationship.

Right now, I'm practicing three times a week, but I wish I had the time to do it every day. I've always thought of yoga as an old reliable friend that will always be there for you. Even if you happen to stray from practicing regularly, it's just a matter of reacquainting yourself with the postures and you're back on track. I've also found that once you start practicing, it becomes a natural part of your life and something that you really look forward to doing.

I initially began yoga for the physical benefits it might offer. The mental relaxation aspect of it was an unexpected benefit I realized a few years later. I worked in high-stress news jobs for a good part of my career, and yoga was instrumental in alleviating some of the constant stress. And I just don't experience any of the aches and pains associated with growing older that I hear about from men my age.

Even though I've been practicing for over 20 years, I would still like to improve my flexibility. And I consider that part of the beauty of yoga: You progress at your own pace. There is no wrong or right rate of progression.

If you're going to give yoga a try, keeping an open mind is critical. Don't go to your first lesson with unrealistic expectations or fear of having to check into some new way of life or religion. Many people hear the word *yoga* and immediately think in terms of something that is antithetical to Judeo-Christian beliefs, but most yoga as it is practiced in the United States is not religious. You must also give yourself time and not be hard on yourself if you can't master a posture on your first attempt.

I think yoga is like swimming. They are both lifelong activities that you can start when you're very young and continue until your last day on Earth. And that is exactly what I intend to do.

Index

Note: Underscored page references indicate boxed text.

Melatonin, 76
Mental acuity, program for
    improving, 92–96, <u>93</u>
Microbrew beers, <u>65</u>
Microscope, development of, 7
Migraine headaches, <u>139</u>
Mind
    in Chinese medicine, <u>93</u>
    functions of
        improving, 92–96, <u>93</u>
        stress on, 96
    healing power of, 38, 40–43,
        <u>41</u>, <u>43</u>
Mind-body connection, 6–7,
    11–13, <u>13</u>, 90
Minerals, healing power of, 68,
    70–71. *See also specific
    minerals*; Supplements
Moisturizers, 110
Monamine oxidase (MAO), 93,
    109, 122
Montezuma's revenge, <u>149</u>
Muscles
    building
        diet for, <u>87</u>
        program for, 86–91, <u>87</u>,
            <u>88–89</u>, <u>91</u>
        supplements for, 72–74, 87
    cramps in, 78
    pubococcygeal, 97–98
    stretching
        exercises, 88–90
        injury prevention and, 88
    tension in, 133
Music therapy
    blood pressure and, lowering,
        124
    brainpower and, improving,
        94–95
    colds and, preventing,
        144–45
    description of, <u>28–29</u>
    flu and, preventing, 144–45
    healing power of, 53–55, <u>55</u>
    immune system and,
        improving, 144–45
    meditation with, 53–54
    national organization for, <u>23</u>
    for relieving
        digestive problems, 150
        headache, 139–40

in stress management, 105–7,
    116–17, 124, 144–45
weight rock room and, <u>88–89</u>
Myelin sheath, 92

N

Nardil, 109
Nasal health, <u>52</u>
National organizations for
    alternative medicine,
    <u>22–23</u>
Native American medicine, 14
Natural cures and preventions,
    for. *See also* Alternative
    medicine; *specific types*
    allergies, 142–43, <u>143</u>
    asthma, 142–43, <u>143</u>
    back pain, 130–33, <u>131</u>, <u>132–33</u>
    bruises, 146–47, <u>147</u>
    cancer, 128–29
    colds, 144–45, <u>145</u>
    cuts, 146–47, <u>147</u>
    digestive problems, 148–50,
        <u>149</u>
    flu, 144–45, <u>145</u>
    headache, 138–41, <u>139</u>,
        <u>140–41</u>
    heart disease, 120–24, <u>121</u>, <u>123</u>
    high cholesterol, 125–27, <u>127</u>
    immunity, boosting, 115–19,
        <u>117</u>, <u>119</u>
    sex problems, 134–37, <u>136–37</u>
Nature Cure, 19
Naturopathy, 19–20, 23, <u>23</u>,
    <u>28–29</u>
Nausea, 150. *See also* Digestive
    problems
Negative thoughts, 41–42
Neuropeptides, 11
Nutrients, 56
Nutrition, 114
Nux vomica, 21

O

Oregano, <u>67</u>
Orgasms, 82
Overland, Kevin, 156–57

P

Pain. *See also* Headache
    arthritis, 76
    back, 80–81, 130–33, <u>131</u>,
        <u>132–33</u>
    dental, 79
    sinus, 78–79, 81, 138
Parsley, <u>67</u>, 112, 146
PC muscle, 97–98
Pectin, 100, 120
Penicillin, 4
Pepotement, 98–99
Peppermint
    in aromatherapy, 50
    for back pain relief, 132
    for digestive problems,
        113
    growing, 32–33
    health benefits of, 114
    tea, 113
Petrissage, 98
Physicians, selecting, 30–31,
    <u>31</u>
Phytochemicals, 56, 120
Pineapple juice, 63
Pisano, Ben, 161
Pitta (fire personality), 18, <u>18</u>
Pizza, 60
Placebo effect, <u>13</u>, 21
Polyphenols, 122–23, 127
Posture, good, 141
Potentizing, 20–21
Poultices, <u>113</u>
Power, healing
    diet, 56–61, <u>57</u>, <u>59</u>, <u>61</u>
    fluid intake, 62–63, <u>63</u>
    hearing, 53–55, <u>55</u>
    herbal medicine, 64–67, <u>65</u>,
        <u>67</u>
    mind, 38, 40–43, <u>41</u>, <u>43</u>
    minerals, 68, 70–71
    path to, 38–39
    sex, 82–84, <u>83</u>
    sight, 46–49, <u>47</u>, <u>48–49</u>
    smell, 51–52, <u>51</u>, <u>52</u>
    spirit, 44–45
    supplements, 71–76, <u>73</u>
    touch, 77–81, <u>79</u>, 81
    vitamins, 68–71, <u>69</u>, <u>71</u>
Prana (life force), 6, 18